Plant-Based Diet

Edited by Blanca Hernández-Ledesma

Published in London, United Kingdom

Plant-Based Diet
http://dx.doi.org/10.5772/intechopen.105283
Edited by Blanca Hernández-Ledesma

Contributors
Imen Ghorbel, Mariem Chaâbane, Naziha Grati Kammoun, Najiba Zeghal, Kuntal Das, Priyabrata Roy, Raj Kumar Singh Tiwari, Mulualem T. T. Kassa, Anteneh T Tefera, Debebe Worku Dadi, Alemayehu Getahun, Asaminew Abiyu, Alphonsus Utioh, Diriba Muleta, Rotimi E. Aluko, Michael S. Donaldson, Ntsoaki Joyce Malebo

First published in London, United Kingdom, 2024 by IntechOpen
IntechOpen is the global imprint of INTECHOPEN LIMITED, registered in England and Wales, registration number: 11086078, 5 Princes Gate Court, London, SW7 2QJ, United Kingdom

British Library Cataloguing-in-Publication Data
A catalogue record for this book is available from the British Library

Additional hard and PDF copies can be obtained from orders@intechopen.com

Plant-Based Diet
Edited by Blanca Hernández-Ledesma
p. cm.
Print ISBN 978-1-83768-952-1
Online ISBN 978-1-83768-953-8
eBook (PDF) ISBN 978-1-83768-954-5

Meet the editor

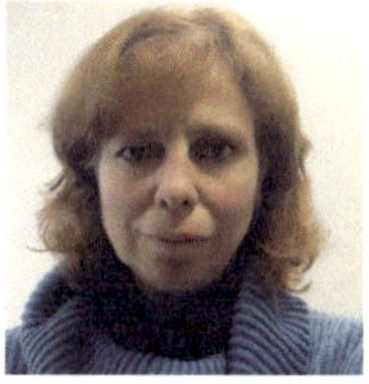

Dr. Hernández-Ledesma is a tenured scientist at the Institute of Food Science Research (CIAL), a joint center of shared ownership between the Higher Council for Scientific Research (CSIC) and the Autonomous University of Madrid (UAM). She developed her distinguished research career in Spain and the United States (University of California, Berkeley). Her current interests are focused on the study of the potential of alternative food sources (vegetables, micro and macroalgae, insects), evaluating the digestibility, bioavailability, and bioactivity of their compounds as the basis for the development of new health-promoting ingredients. She has published more than 100 articles in high-impact scientific journals, 40 book chapters, and several articles in international media. Moreover, she has edited seven books and presented her work at multiple international and national conferences.

Contents

Preface

It is estimated that by 2050 the world's population will exceed 10 billion people, which will lead to a deterioration in global food security. To avoid aggravating this problem, international organizations have recommended dietary changes to reduce animal calorie intake and increase consumption of sustainable, nutrient-rich, calorie-efficient products. In addition, growing awareness of the impact of food on human health and the state of the environment has justified the need to seek alternative sources of food. This has promoted a steady increase in demand for plant-based diets attributed to the growing vegan, vegetarian, and flexitarian population, increasing intolerance to animal proteins, and other factors such as ethical concerns, nutritional benefits of plant-based diets, and increased investments in the plant protein sector. To meet the growing demand for plant-based foods expected over the next decade, there is a need to incorporate new food plant sources that embrace climate-resilient production systems and optimize strategies to increase the yield of improved health-promoting compounds. Moreover, this development must be scientifically documented and efficiently and reliably transferred to the academic world and society, favoring the contribution of all sectors.

The chapters of this book are divided into three sections.

Section 1, "Nutritional Value and Health Benefits of Vegetables", includes three chapters. In Chapter 1 "The Beneficial Role of Nuts and Seeds in a Plant-Based Diet", Michael S. Donaldson aims to answer several questions on the nutritional value of nuts and seeds and their potential health benefits when these plant food sources are incorporated into a plant-based diet. Chapter 2, "African *Moringa stenopetala* Plant: An Emerging Source of Novel Ingredients for Plant-Based Foods", by Anteneh T. Tefera et al., summarizes recent evidence on the potential of this plant, considered a staple food and traditional medicine by the local East African people, as a novel source of ingredients for food, cosmetic, and nutraceutical industries. Similarly, in Chapter 3 "Nutritional and Functional Value of African Leafy Vegetables: Advantages and Limitations", Ntsoaki Joyce Malebo shows the advantages of the consumption of African leafy vegetables as an alternative food source because of their high nutritional value and health properties. This chapter also summarizes the limitations associated with the intake of these plant sources due to their perishable character, low bioavailability of some bioactive compounds, and low acceptability by current consumers.

Section 2, "Bioactive Compounds from Vegetal Sources", includes Chapter 4, "Beneficial Effects of Extra Virgin Olive Oil Rich in Phenolic Compounds on Cardiovascular Health". In this chapter, Imen Ghorbel et al. clarify the beneficial effect of extra virgin olive oil on cardiovascular risk factors when included as part of the Mediterranean diet, and review the basic mechanisms by which the polyphenols present in this oil exert their activities.

Finally, Section 3, “Strategies for Nutritional Security”, includes one chapter written by Kuntal Das et al. Chapter 5, “Biofortification of Rice, An Impactful Strategy for Nutritional Security: Current Perspectives and Future Prospect”, discusses the advantages and challenges of rice biofortification as a strategy to improve human nutritional security. It also summarizes the dissemination among stakeholders and trends in acceptance by consumers.

In conclusion, this book is intended to assist and guide food scientists, engineers, and nutritionists working in the field of food science, as well as consumers who are aware of the need to adopt healthy and low environmental impact dietary patterns.

I would like to take this opportunity to thank all the authors who have participated in this book for their cooperation and the quality of their work. Editing this book has allowed me to interact with prestigious researchers from different countries such as the United States, Canada, China, India, South Africa, Ethiopia, and Tunisia.

Blanca Hernández-Ledesma
Institute of Food Science Research (CIAL, CSIC-UAM),
Madrid, Spain

Section 1

Nutritional Value and Health Benefits of Vegetables

Chapter 1

The Beneficial Role of Nuts and Seeds in a Plant-Based Diet

Michael S. Donaldson

Abstract

In the last several years research has been accumulating that demonstrates that nuts and seeds are beneficial for all people. While some plant-based diet programs have embraced the inclusion of nuts and seeds, other programs have eschewed nuts and seeds, remaining firmly committed to a starch-based dietary pattern. This chapter assembles the scientific evidence regarding the benefits of nuts and seeds into three issues: (1) The nutrient density of nuts and seeds compared to grains and legumes of the same caloric content, (2) The improvement of health outcomes and extra benefits when nuts and seeds are included in plant-based diets, (3) The safety of nuts and seeds when a person is dealing with cancer. As a result of examining these issues with the known scientific evidence it will become apparent that one to two ounces of nuts and seeds daily is a very beneficial part of a plant-based diet.

Keywords: nuts, seeds, cardiovascular disease, cancer, plant based diet

1. Introduction

The scientific evidence for the benefits of a plant-based diet is enumerated in the various chapters of this book. Much of the evidence comes from programs and clinical trials that avoided any added fats or fatty foods, even from plant sources. So a title containing "nuts" and "benefits" in the same sentence may seem like an oxymoron, a contradiction in terms at the least. The inclusion of fatty foods like nuts and seeds has been and continues to be a controversial topic within the plant-based research community. While newer publications from the last several years relate to benefits of nuts and seeds, the older plant-based diet literature largely found positive results without the inclusion of nuts or seeds. Dr. Dean Ornish and Dr. Caldwell Esselstyn established the benefits of a low-fat plant-based diet for reversing heart disease. Dr. Ornish was one of the first doctors to prove that a plant-based diet could reverse heart disease, using the best testing methods available to provide the evidence to sway beliefs [1]. Dr. Esselstyn also reversed heart disease using this very low-fat diet, having about a 99% success rate [2]. Both Dr. Ornish and Dr. Esselstyn were able to get their great clinical success purposefully avoiding nuts and seeds and any added fats in the diet. Their success has been continued by others as well [3].

On the other hand, the position paper of the American Dietetic Association states "A well-planned vegetarian diet containing vegetables, fruits, whole grains, legumes, nuts, and seeds can provide adequate nutrition." [4]. The use of enhanced intake of beans, greens, seeds, nuts, whole grains, and other colorful plant products is recommended for athletes by Fuhrman and Ferreri [5]. In examining protein intakes on plant-based diets Mariotti and Gardner warn, "An insufficient protein intake from vegetarian diets may occur if the diet does not include protein-rich foods such as legumes (the most traditional source) and nuts and seeds, or any protein analogs of animal foods" [6].

In view of the lingering scientific controversy of the inclusion of nuts and seeds into a healthy plant-based diet this chapter is written so that the information is clearly available in one place for people to understand how nuts and seeds can be beneficial. There are 3 main issues to be addressed in this article. They are:

1. The nutrient density of nuts and seeds compared to grains and legumes.

2. The improvement of health outcomes and extra benefits when nuts and seeds are included in vegetarian or vegan diets.

3. The safety of nuts and seeds when a person is dealing with cancer.

As a result of examining these issues, it will become apparent that 1 to 2 ounces of nuts and seeds on a daily basis is a very beneficial part of a healthy plant-based diet.

2. Nutrient density of nuts versus grains and legumes

The first issue is to examine the nutrient density of nuts and seeds compared to grains and legumes. To examine this issue, four common nuts and five common seeds were compared with five grains and six types of beans and lentils. A 200-calorie serving of each food was compared for nutrients, as this is just slightly more than a 1 ounce serving of nuts or seeds. Nutrient amounts were taken from USDA standard reference nutrient tables incorporated into the software program NutriBase (Version 11.71, Phoenix, AZ).

As shown in **Table 1**, equal caloric amounts of nuts, cooked grains and cooked beans vary in serving sizes, measured in grams. About 1 ounce of seeds or nuts yields 200 calories, while it takes about one cup of cooked grains or about ¾ cup of cooked beans to get the same amount of calories. The main difference is the amount of water that is not in nuts and seeds and the fact that fats pack more calories into a smaller space than carbohydrates and proteins.

2.1 Macronutrient content in nuts versus grains and legumes

Nuts and seeds and grains have about 6.5 grams of protein per 200-calorie serving, while cooked dry beans have about double this amount, at 13 grams of protein per 200-calorie serving. So for protein, beans are a better source of protein than nuts and seeds. Beans average 35% of the calories as protein, ranging from 26 percent (pink beans and chickpeas) to 40 percent (lentils). Nuts and seeds are about 14% protein, ranging from about 5 percent (pecans) to 20 percent (pumpkin seed kernels). Grains are similar to nuts in protein content ranging from 10 percent (brown rice) to 16 percent (quinoa).

Ingredient	Grams	Protein (g)	%Cal, Protein	Carbs (g)	Fiber (g)	Net Carb (g)	%Cal, Carb	Fat (g)	%Cal, Fat
Almond, Raw	35.0	7.3	14.8	7.5	4.3	3.1	6.4	17.3	78.8
Walnut, Raw	30.6	4.7	9.0	4.2	2.1	2.2	4.2	20.0	86.8
Pecan, Raw	29.0	2.7	5.2	4.0	2.8	1.2	2.4	20.9	92.3
Pistachio, Rstd	35.3	7.4	14.8	10.4	3.5	6.9	13.8	15.8	71.4
Sunflower Seed	34.3	7.1	14.0	6.9	3.0	3.9	7.7	17.7	78.3
Sesame Seed	34.9	6.2	12.6	8.2	4.1	4.1	8.3	17.3	79.2
Flax Seed	37.5	6.9	15.9	10.8	10.2	0.6	1.4	15.8	82.7
Chia Seed	41.2	6.8	17.7	17.4	14.2	3.2	8.3	12.7	74.0
Pumpkin Seed	35.8	10.8	20.8	3.8	2.2	1.7	3.2	17.6	76.0
Nuts & Seeds, Average	**34.8**	**6.7**	**13.9**	**8.1**	**5.1**	**3.0**	**6.2**	17.2	79.9
Quinoa, ckd	166.7	7.3	16.2	35.5	4.7	30.8	68.0	3.2	15.9
Wild Rice, ckd	198	7.9	16.4	42.3	3.6	38.7	80.4	0.7	3.2
Brown Rice, ckd	180.2	4.7	10.0	41.4	3.2	38.1	82.1	1.6	7.9
WW Bread	72.0	6.0	12.7	37.0	4.3	32.7	68.8	3.9	18.4
Oatmeal, wtr	281.7	7.2	15.6	33.8	4.8	29.0	63.3	4.3	21.0
Grains, Average	**179.7**	**6.6**	**14.2**	38.0	**4.1**	33.9	72.5	**2.7**	**13.3**
Pinto Bean, bld	139.9	12.6	32.5	36.7	12.6	24.1	62.2	0.9	5.3
Black Bean, bld	151.5	13.4	35.3	35.9	13.2	22.7	59.8	0.8	4.8
Chickpea, cnd	227.3	11.2	26.7	30.7	10.0	20.7	49.4	4.4	23.9
GN Bean, bld	169.5	14.1	35.6	35.8	11.9	23.9	60.1	0.8	4.3
Navy Bean, bld	142.9	11.8	32.7	37.2	15.0	22.2	61.8	0.9	5.5
Pink Bean, bld	134.2	12.2	27.6	37.5	7.1	30.3	69.0	0.7	3.4
Lentil, bld	172.4	15.6	40.8	34.7	13.6	21.1	55.3	0.7	3.9
Beans, Average	**162.5**	13.0	33.0	**35.5**	11.9	**23.6**	**59.7**	**1.3**	**7.3**

Food group with the highest amount of a nutrient shown in red. Rstd = roasted; Bld = boiled; Ckd = cooked; WW = whole wheat; wtr = prepared with water; cnd = canned; GN Bean = Great Northern Bean.

Table 1.
Proximate nutrient comparison of 200 calories servings of nuts, grains and dry beans.

Carbohydrate content is again a big difference between nuts and seeds and grains/beans. The carbohydrate content of nuts and seeds is very low, especially considering their fiber content. Nuts and seeds averaged about 3 grams of net carbohydrate per 200-calorie serving. Only pistachios were above 5 grams. Grains averaged about 34 grams of net carbs, while beans averaged 24 grams. About 72% of the calories in grains come from carbohydrates; 60% of calories in beans are from carbohydrates.

Fiber is another category where the beans are about double the amount in nuts and seeds and grains, with about 12 grams of fiber per serving of beans compared to about 4 grams for grains and 5 grams for nuts and seeds. Flax seeds and chia seeds are much higher in fiber than other seeds or nuts. The average fiber content without these two seeds is 3.1 grams per serving.

Nuts and seeds are rich in fat, with about 80 percent of the calories coming from fats. Pecans and walnuts are particularly high in fat, with 87 and 92 percent of their calories, respectively, coming from fat. Beans on average have about 4.5 percent of the calories as fat, except for chickpeas which are at about 24 percent. Grains are also naturally low in fat.

So, nuts and seeds are a modest source of protein, very low in carbohydrates and a rich source of fats. Grains are a modest source of protein, low in fat and have a large amount of starch in them. Dry beans and lentils are an excellent source of protein, very low in fat, and a very good source of fiber as well.

One of the benefits of nuts and seeds here is the lack of glycemic response from their consumption. A recent randomized trial compared glucose and insulin levels after consuming a 253-calorie serving of mixed nuts or unsalted pretzels after an overnight fast. In the pretzel group glucose and insulin levels 60 minutes after eating were elevated, while in the mixed nuts group neither glucose nor insulin levels were significantly different from baseline levels [7]. In addition to nuts, flax seeds and chia seeds are very rich in dietary fiber. When 15 volunteers took, in random order, a 50-gram glucose challenge by itself or along with 25 g chia seeds or 31.5 g flax seeds the blood glucose response during 2 hours was blunted significantly by 39 and 28% by chia seeds and flax seeds, respectively [8]. These seeds, especially chia seeds, were able to turn glucose into a slow-release carbohydrate with their high-viscosity fiber.

A comparison of the classes of fats in nuts and seeds is given in **Figure 1** for a 200-calorie serving of four kinds of nuts and five kinds of seeds. As seen in **Figure 1**, there is very little saturated fat in nuts and seeds. Almonds, pecans, and pistachio nuts are high in monounsaturated fatty acids (MUFAs) with over 50 percent of their fat as MUFA. Only walnuts, flax seeds, and chia seeds have significant amounts of omega 3 polyunsaturated fatty acids (PUFAs) as alpha linolenic acid (ALA), a short-chain omega 3 fatty acid. Walnuts, sunflower, sesame, and pumpkin seeds have a large amount of the omega 6 fatty acid linoleic acid (LA). In their unprocessed, raw form both LA and ALA are very valuable fats and are essential nutrients, not found in grains and legumes in appreciable amounts. This is another benefit of nuts and seeds. So, these raw nuts and seeds are a good source of LA and ALA, which can be damaged by roasting, especially for long times over the temperature of 300°F (150°C) [9]. Though only trace amounts are transformed into the long-chain omega 3 fatty acid DHA [10], there are many health benefits from ALA and EPA generated from ALA [11]. Overall, the fatty acid profiles of nuts and seeds are very favorable to cardiovascular health as MUFAs and especially PUFAs tend to lower cholesterol and the incidence of cardiovascular disease compared to saturated fats [12]. And whatever is protective of the heart is likely to be beneficial for the brain, bones, joints, and muscles of the body.

2.2 Vitamin content

A comparison of the vitamin content of 200-calorie servings of common nuts and seeds, grains and dry beans is given in **Table 2**. The Recommended Daily Intake (RDI) is given for each nutrient, as it is much easier to compare percentages rather than actual amounts. The nutrient amount for a particular food is in bold case for amounts greater than 20 percent of the RDI. As you can see, these foods are not a rich source of several of these vitamins, such as vitamin A, vitamin C, and vitamin K. These vitamins are found in higher amounts in fruits and vegetables. The vitamins which contents are high in nuts and seeds are mentioned in the text below.

DOI: http://dx.doi.org/10.5772/intechopen.110677

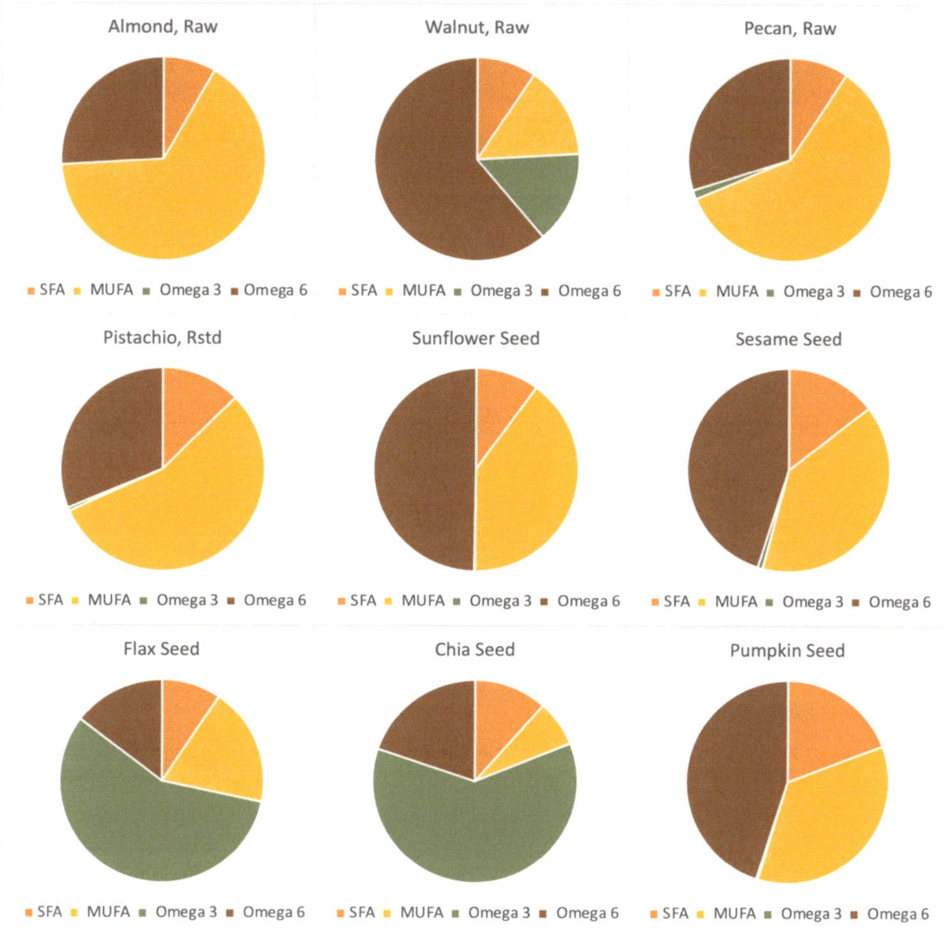

Figure 1.
A breakdown of the distribution of saturated, monounsaturated and polyunsaturated fats in nuts and seeds. SFA = saturated fat, MUFA = monounsaturated fat, Omega 3 = alpha linolenic acid, Omega 6 = linoleic acid.

Ingredient	Vit-A µg RAE	B1 mg	B2 mg	B3 mg	B5 mg	B6 mg	Chol mg	Folate µg DFE	Vit C mg	Vit E mg	K1 µg
RDI, absolute amounts	900	1.2	1.3	16	5	1.7	550	400	90	15	120
Almond, Raw	0%	6%	**30%**	8%	3%	3%	3%	4%	0%	**59%**	0%
Walnut, Raw	0%	8%	4%	2%	3%	9%	2%	7%	0%	1%	1%
Pecan, Raw	0.1%	16%	3%	2%	5%	4%	2%	2%	0%	3%	1%
Pistachio, Rstd	0.5%	**21%**	6%	3%	4%	**24%**	5%	5%	1%	6%	4%
Sunflower Seed	0.1%	**43%**	9%	18%	8%	**27%**	3%	19%	1%	**80%**	0%
Sesame Seed	0%	**23%**	7%	10%	0%	16%	2%	8%	0%	1%	0%
Flax Seed	0%	**52%**	5%	7%	7%	11%	5%	8%	0%	1%	1%
Chia Seed	0%	**22%**	5%	**23%**					1%	1%	
Pumpkin Seed	0%	8%	4%	11%	5%	3%	4%	5%	1%	5%	2%

Ingredient	Vit-A µg RAE	B1 mg	B2 mg	B3 mg	B5 mg	B6 mg	Chol mg	Folate µg DFE	Vit C mg	Vit E mg	K1 µg
Nuts & Seeds, Average	0.1%	**22%**	8%	9%	5%	12%	3%	7%	0%	17%	1%
Quinoa, ckd	0%	15%	14%	4%		12%	7%	18%	0%	7%	0%
Wild Rice, ckd	0%	8%	13%	16%	6%	16%	4%	13%	0%	3%	1%
Brown Rice, ckd	0%	14%	4%	17%	10%	15%	3%	2%	0%	0%	1%
WW Bread	0%	18%	12%	18%	7%	8%	3%	14%	0%	4%	6%
Oatmeal, wtr	0%	18%	3%	4%	18%	1%	4%	4%	0%	2%	1%
Grains, Average	0%	15%	9%	12%	10%	10%	4%	10%	0%	3%	2%
Pinto Bean, bld	0%	**23%**	7%	3%	6%	19%		**60%**	1%	9%	4%
Black Bean, bld	0%	**31%**	7%	5%	7%	6%		**56%**	0%	0%	0%
Chickpea, cnd	0.2%	6%	2%	2%	14%	**63%**	10%	14%	0%	3%	4%
GN Bean, bld	0%	**23%**	8%	7%	9%	12%		**43%**	2%		
Navy Bean, bld	0%	**28%**	7%	6%	8%	12%	12%	**50%**		0%	1%
Pink Bean, bld	0%	**28%**	6%	5%	8%	14%	9%	**56%**	0%	9%	4%
Lentil, bld	0.1%	**24%**	10%	11%	**22%**	18%	10%	**78%**	3%	1%	2%
Beans, Average	**0%**	23%	7%	6%	10%	**21%**	**10%**	**51%**	1%	4%	3%

Excellent sources of nutrients (≥ 20% of RDI) are shown in bold case. Blank cells indicate missing data. Rstd = roasted; Bld = boiled; Ckd = cooked; WW = whole wheat; wtr = prepared with water; cnd = canned; GN Bean = Great Northern Bean.

Table 2.
Vitamin comparison of nuts, grains and dry beans, as a percent of the recommended dietary intake (RDI).

A serving of sunflower seeds provides over 40 percent of the RDI for thiamin (vitamin B1). A 200-calorie serving of flax seeds provides over 50 percent of the RDI. Most seeds are generally an excellent source of thiamin, with pumpkin seeds being the exception. Grains on average provide 15 percent of the RDI. Beans are also an excellent source of vitamin B1, providing between 20 and 30 percent of the RDI for thiamin, similar to the average for seeds.

A serving of almonds provides over 30 percent of the RDI for riboflavin (vitamin B2). But most nuts and seeds are not this rich a source of riboflavin, averaging about 5 percent of the RDI. Grains and beans are not much better, with less than 10 percent of the RDI per serving.

Sunflowers are a notable source of niacin (vitamin B3), with 18 percent of the RDI per serving. But chia seeds are even better at 23 percent. Rice and whole wheat bread are good sources with 16–18 percent of the RDI of niacin per serving. Beans are not a rich source of niacin with only lentils providing more than 10 percent of the RDI.

Pistachio nuts and sunflower seeds are excellent sources of vitamin B6, with sesame and flax seeds also being good sources. Grains are good sources, except for oatmeal. Beans are also good sources, with chickpeas delivering over 60% of the RDI per serving.

Almonds and sunflower seeds are very rich sources of vitamin E. Most other nuts and seeds, grains and beans provide little vitamin E, but these two foods are two of the richest food sources of vitamin E. In a South Korean trial using 56 g/day of almonds or a control cookie in a 4-week cross-over pattern, volunteers doubled their intake of vitamin E, which resulted in an 8.5% increase in plasma α-tocopherol levels while simultaneously reducing total cholesterol 5.5% and non-HDL cholesterol by 6.4% [13].

From this analysis of vitamins, we can deduce a few points. First, different foods have different strengths as sources of nutrients, so it is helpful to encourage people to eat a variety of plant foods to take advantage of different nutrient profiles to even out overall intake. Second, when averaging the percent of the RDI for each vitamin, sunflower seeds are, on average, the best source of micronutrients (19%) of all of these foods listed in **Table 3**. Almonds are also a good source of vitamins with an

Ingredient	Calc (mg)	Mag (mg)	Phos (mg)	Pot (mg)	Cop (mg)	Iron (mg)	Mng (mg)	Sel (μg)	Zn (mg)
RDI, absolute amounts	1300	420	1250	4700	0.9	18	2.3	55	11
Almond, Raw	7%	**22%**	13%	5%	**40%**	7%	**33%**	3%	10%
Walnut, Raw	2%	12%	8%	3%	**54%**	5%	**45%**	3%	9%
Pecan, Raw	2%	8%	6%	3%	**39%**	4%	**57%**	2%	12%
Pistachio, Rstd	3%	9%	13%	8%	**51%**	8%	19%	6%	8%
Sunflower Seed	2%	**27%**	18%	5%	**69%**	10%	**29%**	33%	16%
Sesame Seed	**26%**	**29%**	18%	3%	**69%**	28%	**37%**	22%	**25%**
Flax Seed	7%	**35%**	19%	6%	**51%**	12%	**40%**	17%	15%
Chia Seed	**20%**	**33%**	**28%**	4%	**42%**	18%	**49%**	41%	17%
Pumpkin Seed	1%	**33%**	**35%**	6%	**53%**	18%	**71%**	6%	**25%**
Nuts & Seeds, Average	8%	**25%**	18%	5%	**62%**	12%	**42%**	15%	15%
Quinoa, ckd	2%	**25%**	**20%**	6%	**36%**	14%	**46%**	8%	17%
Wild Rice, ckd	0%	15%	13%	4%	**27%**	7%	**24%**	3%	**24%**
Brown Rice, ckd	1%	18%	12%	2%	**20%**	4%	**71%**	**32%**	10%
WW Bread	2%	14%	11%	5%	**20%**	12%	**59%**	**50%**	10%
Oatmeal, wtr	2%	18%	17%	4%	**23%**	14%	**71%**	**28%**	**26%**
Grains, Average	2%	18%	15%	4%	**25%**	10%	**54%**	**24%**	17%
Pinto Bean, bld	5%	17%	16%	13%	**34%**	16%	**27%**	16%	12%
Black Bean, bld	3%	25%	17%	11%	**36%**	18%	**29%**	3%	15%
Chickpea, cnd	6%	15%	15%	7%	**39%**	16%	**81%**	8%	14%
GN Bean, bld	9%	20%	**22%**	14%	**47%**	20%	**81%**	13%	14%
Navy Bean, bld	8%	18%	16%	12%	**33%**	19%	**33%**	8%	13%
Pink Bean, bld	5%	21%	18%	15%	**40%**	17%	**33%**	3%	12%
Lentil, bld	3%	15%	**25%**	14%	**48%**	32%	**37%**	9%	**20%**
Beans, Average	6%	19%	18%	12%	**40%**	20%	**40%**	9%	14%

Table 3.
Mineral Comparison of Nuts, Grains and Dry Beans, as a Percent of the Recommended Dietary Intake (RDI). Excellent sources of nutrients (≥ 20% of RDI) are shown in bold case.

average of 11% RDI. Beans average is 12% RDI, with lentils coming in highest at 16%. This vitamin analysis shows that sunflower seeds, almonds, and lentils are great foods for at least weekly consumption, if not more frequently.

2.3 Mineral content

As can be seen from **Table 3**, nuts and seeds, whole grains and dry beans all provide a much higher amount of the essential minerals than of the vitamins. The RDI amount in milligrams or micrograms (for selenium) are given in the first row of the table.

Sesame seeds and chia seeds are both excellent sources of calcium, providing 26 and 20 percent of the RDI, respectively. Almonds and flax seeds are also decent sources, with about 95 mg of calcium per serving. Great Northern beans and navy beans are also decent sources of calcium, around 100 mg per serving, but the other beans are not so high. Calcium has long been a nutrient of concern for people following plant-based diets, so the inclusion of nuts and seeds rich in calcium will boost intakes of calcium compared to eating isocaloric amounts of grains.

Magnesium is a shortfall nutrient for the US population. About 50 percent of all American consume less than the Estimated Average Requirement (EAR) for magnesium [14]. Among the elderly it is worse, with 75% of men age 71+ and 63% of women age 71+ under the EAR for magnesium. Adolescents do not fare well, either, with 78 and 89 percent of males and females, respectively, 14–18 years of age consuming less than the EAR. Magnesium is very important for cardiovascular health, bone health, prevention of diabetes, cognitive function [15], and prevention of eclampsia during pregnancy [16].

Consuming more nuts and seeds can improve intake of magnesium. On average nuts and seeds are better sources of magnesium than grains or beans, though there is some variation. A 200-calorie serving of seeds averages 35% of the RDI for magnesium, making them a superfood for magnesium. Almonds are the only nut that is an excellent source (≥20% of RDI) of magnesium. Grains are good sources, with quinoa excelling at 25% of RDI for magnesium. Some beans are excellent sources of magnesium (black beans, Great Northern beans, pink beans) and the average for beans comes out to 18% of RDI for magnesium. Generally, grains and beans have only half of the amount of magnesium found in seeds, so substituting a serving of seeds for a serving of whole grains will improve a persons' magnesium status.

Though high intake of potassium is a strength of plant-based diets and contributes to normal blood pressure [17], strong bones [18], and cardiovascular and overall survival [19], nuts and seeds and grains are low sources of potassium, while beans are generally good sources. Potassium is found in abundance in fruit and vegetables, so this is where most of the requirements are met. Beans win this mineral by a two-fold margin.

Copper is easily obtained in a plant-based diet. It is easy to get half of the RDI for copper with a 200-calorie serving of nuts or seeds. Sesame seeds provide 1.4 mg of copper, almost 160% of the RDI. Beans are also an excellent source of copper, but not as good as nuts and seeds.

Plant-based diets need good sources of iron. Women of reproductive age following plant-based diets especially need iron to replace iron lost in their monthly reproductive cycle to prevent anemia. While some whole grains are good sources of iron, seeds are an even better source of iron, and sesame seeds are an excellent source. Nuts and rice are not rich in iron. Beans are a good source, with lentils and Great Northern beans being excellent sources. Beans, on average, are a better source of iron than even the seeds.

Selenium is important as an antioxidant mineral, contributing to the synthesis of the intracellular antioxidant glutathione and selenoproteins. Good selenium status has been found to improve a body's defenses against viral diseases such as HIV and COVID [20]. Brazil nuts are well known for their selenium content, a listing of over 580 μg per 200 calories (30.5 grams, about 6 nuts). Other nuts are generally low in selenium along with beans, but most seeds are an excellent source of selenium. Pinto beans and Great Northern beans are good sources of selenium.

Zinc is an essential mineral with many roles in the body. Zinc plays a role in immune defense, showing effectiveness against respiratory viruses [21]. Higher dietary intake of zinc from non-red meat sources was associated with lower risk of progression of coronary artery calcification scores [22]. Nuts and seeds are generally good sources of zinc, with sesame seeds and pumpkin seeds being excellent sources. Wild rice and oatmeal, but not whole wheat, are also excellent sources of zinc from the grain category. Dry beans are good sources, with lentils being an excellent source of zinc.

In conclusion, when averaging the RDIs for all minerals, nuts have 15%, seeds have 28%, grains 19% and beans 20% of the RDIs. So, nuts are not as mineral dense as seeds, but seeds are a really good way of increasing essential mineral intake. Overall mineral intake is important, as indicated in a study of the Iowa Women's Health Study. Quintiles of mineral intake were used to create an overall mineral score, with positive scores for calcium, magnesium, manganese, zinc, selenium, potassium and iodine, and negative scores for iron, copper, phosphorus and sodium. Higher ranks of the mineral score were associated with lower risk of colorectal cancer in these 55- to 69-year-old women, up to 25% decreased risk comparing highest to lowest rank of mineral score [23]. So, increasing mineral intake by substituting a serving of grains out for a serving of seeds will likely reduce risk of disease.

2.4 Summary of nutrient comparison

To summarize this section nuts and seeds are the category of food that is the best way to get an extra 200 calories. When comparing just nuts and seeds versus grains one can see that nuts and seeds are more nutrient dense and deliver more nutrients per 200 calories. The average percentage of RDI for vitamins and minerals are 14.4 percent for nuts and seeds and 12.3 percent for grains (see **Table 4**). However, if we remove walnuts, pecans and pistachio nuts from the equation and just look at almonds

Food Group	Average % of RDI	Nutrient Density
Grains	12.3%	1.0
All nuts and seeds	14.4%	+17%
Beans	15.6%	+27%
Almonds and seeds	17.6%	+43%
Seeds	18.5%	+50%
Lentils	19.1%	+55%

Table 4.
Summary of comparison of nutrient density of food groups.

and the seeds, the average RDI is now 17.6 percent. This is 43 percent more nutrition than what you get from grains, on average. So, seeds and almonds are more nutrient dense than grains.

When comparing nuts and seeds versus beans it can be seen that almonds and seeds have a slightly higher average RDI compared to the beans (17.6 versus 15.6 percent). So, even though they are lower in protein (about 7.5 versus 13 g of protein per serving) almonds and seeds are still overall more nutritionally dense than the average dry bean. For some nutrients beans, especially lentils, are actually more nutrient dense, so it would be wise to still be include beans in the diet as well, but not in the place of a serving of nuts and/or seeds.

So, it can be concluded that nuts, particularly almonds, and seeds are nutritionally more dense than grains, about 43 percent more. Seeds are also about 19 percent more nutritionally dense than dry beans in general. Should almonds and seeds replace grains in this 200-calorie serving? From a nutrient standpoint the answer is a clear yes.

3. Health outcomes of eating nuts and seeds

As mentioned in the introduction, Drs. Esselstyn and Ornish obtained excellent results in reversing heart disease without the inclusion of nuts and seeds. However, since the publication of their results there have been many investigations in the area of nuts and seeds. There have been short-term studies on the effects of various nuts on cholesterol and blood lipids. There have been short-term studies on satiety and weight loss and/or weight gain. There have been prospective cohort studies that have reported observations of groups of people over long periods of time. And there have been some randomized controlled clinical trials using nuts and seeds as well. Now we have more evidence about the benefits of nuts and seeds.

The issue to be examined here is whether health outcomes are better or worse when nuts and seeds are included in vegetarian or vegan diets.

This issue will be examined from four lines of evidence: (1) short-term studies on weight gain and obesity, (2) short-term studies on blood lipids, (3) health outcomes in population studies, and (4) vegetarian population studies in particular.

3.1 Short-term body weight studies

Since nuts are energy-dense foods, it is important to know if they caused weight gain, or if they were associated with obesity. In a review and meta-analysis of 33 controlled clinical trials, it was found there was no difference in body weight, body mass index (BMI) or waist circumference between the nut or control diet groups [24]. Population studies have also found that nut consumption did not affect body weight. People who regularly ate nuts actually tended to not gain weight or become obese over time [25, 26]. It appears that people compensate for eating nuts by eating less of other foods. Nuts' fat and protein content tend to make them a satisfying, filling food, whether eaten as snacks or with meals [27].

3.2 Short-term blood lipid studies

Since population studies have indicated that nuts reduced risk of cardiovascular disease, short-term studies have been conducted to attempt to deduce the mechanism for this health outcome. Many controlled clinical trials have examined different nuts and blood lipid levels, but there are few reports including inflammatory markers and endothelial function. A review and meta-analysis of 61 blood lipid studies found that for a 1-ounce (28 gram) serving of nuts per day, there was a decrease in total cholesterol (−4.7 mg/dL), low-density lipoprotein (LDL) cholesterol (−4.8 mg/dL), ApoB lipoprotein (−3.7 mg/dL) and triglycerides (−2.2 mg/dL) [28]. The results were better for 2 ounces a day than for just 1 daily ounce. This significant, but small decrease in cholesterol levels is probably not the only reason that nuts are beneficial, but these results do point in the right direction. A recent review of 26 walnut controlled interventions found similar results, with no negative effects on body weight or blood pressure [29]. Almonds have been examined separately as well, with 27 almond-control datasets yielding very similar results [30]. So, the amount of nuts rather than the type of nut contributes to the lipid-lowering effect.

Studies have also examined the effect of nuts on blood pressure. No consistent significant results have been obtained [31]. Nor have there been significant reductions in markers of inflammation. Serum C-reactive protein has been measured in multiple studies with little change due to eating nuts [32].

However, there has been a consistent improvement in endothelial cell function, measured by flow-mediated dilation (FMD). Endothelial cells allow more blood flow through the release of nitric oxide. Flow-mediated dilation is a strong predictor of future cardiovascular disease [33]. A review of 10 trials found that nut consumption significantly improved FMD, but walnuts were the only nut that had a significant effect [34].

In summary, short-term studies have found significant effects on cholesterol levels, and walnuts for endothelial function, but no significant effects for blood pressure or inflammation. Nuts also contain phytosterols and other antioxidants that may be beneficial. Whatever the mechanism, long-term studies of populations of people have clearly demonstrated an advantage of eating nuts and seeds.

3.3 Long-term studies of populations

A recent review of reviews and meta-analyses on nuts and cardiovascular disease was published. There have been so many studies and meta-analyses of studies, which synthesize the information from individual studies into a coherent conclusive statement, that they could actually do an overview of all of the reviews and meta-analyses that have been done on population studies of eating nuts. There are 234 references to reviews, meta-analyses and large individual study reports in this article by Kim et al. [35]. Here is what these authors found about nuts and cardiometabolic disease. Consumption of nuts was associated with a 19–20 percent decrease in all-cause mortality. Coronary heart disease (CHD) incidence was reduced by 20–34 percent and CHD death was reduced by 27–30 percent. Cardiovascular disease (CVD) incidence (includes strokes as well as heart disease) was reduced by 19 percent and CVD death was reduced by 25 percent. Stroke incidence was reduced by 10–11 percent and stroke death was reduced by 18 percent.

In addition to this review, Aune et al. [36] have found a 15 percent reduction in total cancer death and a 39 percent decrease in diabetes deaths, and a 75 percent decrease in infectious disease deaths. For specific cancers, Wu et al. [37] reviewed 36 observational studies with a total of over 30,000 people. They found significant associations between eating nuts and a 15 percent overall reduction in cancer. Specific cancers with reductions were colorectal cancer (24% reduction), endometrial cancer (42% reduction), and pancreatic cancer (32% reduction). A recent meta-analysis by

Naghshi et al. [38], which included 43 articles on cancer risk and 9 articles on cancer mortality, found a 14% reduction in cancer risk associated with total nut intake, and a 13% reduction in overall cancer mortality from eating nuts, in close agreement with the work of Aune et al. [36]. A 5 g/d increase in nut intake was found to be associated with a 3, 6 and 25% lower risk of overall, pancreatic and colon cancer, respectively.

It is possible that the people eating nuts are just healthier overall because of other dietary choices and lifestyle habits. Even though population studies control for other dietary and lifestyle factors, there is a small question still. Direct evidence against the healthy nut eater hypothesis comes from a population study from Iran. In the 50,000-person Golestan Cohort nut eating was not associated with other healthy lifestyle habits. People who ate more nuts were also more likely to smoke, drink alcohol, be obese, less likely to exercise, but also were younger, of higher social economic status and had more education. In this cohort the nuts were still protective, leading to less coronary heart disease death and cancer death, especially among women. All-cause mortality was 29 percent less among people consuming three or more servings of nuts per week [39]. So, it appears that the benefits of nuts can be attributed to the nuts consumption and not to other lifestyle behaviors.

3.4 Long-term studies of vegetarian populations

The benefits of nuts have been seen among vegetarians and vegans who have healthy lifestyles as well. In a publication from the Adventist Health Study 2, there was a factor analysis looking at the sources of protein and risk of death [40]. For animal protein, there was a 61 percent increased risk of cardiovascular death, but for the nut protein factor there was a 40 percent decrease in risk of cardiovascular death. There were no significant associations with the factors for protein from grains, processed foods, or legumes, fruits, and vegetables. Among younger adults, aged 25–44 the meat protein factor risk was associated with 2-fold higher risk of cardiovascular death and the nut factor was associated with 3-fold lower risk. Nuts seemed to be protective and meat protein specifically seemed to increase risk of death. The protective effect of nuts was seen across different levels of plant-based dietary patterns in this population, suggesting that focusing on more specific plant protein-based diets may improve the ability of dietary recommendations to prevent CVD.

In the first Adventist Health Study this protective effect of nuts was first reported. When people who ate nuts at least 4 times per week were compared to those who ate nuts less than 1 time per week there was a 48 percent decrease in fatal CHD events and a 55 percent decrease in definite non-fatal heart attacks in the nut-eating group [41]. This protective effect was seen regardless of sex, age, smoking status, hypertensive status, vegetarian or nonvegetarian, exercise level, or whether or not people ate white bread. Nuts were protective despite all these other factors.

3.5 Summary of health benefits of nuts and seeds

The health benefits of nuts and seeds are summarized in **Table 5**. The evidence is robust. The benefits of nuts have been seen in at least 20 different cohorts, including populations at least from the USA, Europe, Iran, and China over a period of more than 26 years. The benefits from one or two ounces of nuts per day are substantial —20% reduction in all-cause mortality, 30% reduction in death by heart disease, 18% reduction in stroke death, 39% reduction in type 2 diabetes death and a 13–15% reduction in

Description of Study	Amount of Nuts	Study Length	Health Outcomes	Ref.
n = 1888, 33 clinical trials	Varied	Varied	No significant difference in body weight, BMI, waist circumference	Flores-Mateo [24]
n = 51,188 women, Nurses' Health Study II	≥2 X /wk. vs. rare	8 years	Slightly less weight gain over time, non-significant lower risk of obesity	Bes-Rastrollo [25]
n = 373,293, EPIC-PANACEA	12.4 g/d median vs. none	5 years	↓5% becoming overweight or obese	Freisling 2018 [26]
Meta-analysis of 61 controlled clinical studies, n = 2852	1 serving = 28 g/d Median dose 56 g/d	3 to 26 weeks	Nut intake (per serving/d) lowered total cholesterol −4.7 mg/dL, LDL cholesterol −4.8 mg/dL, ApoB -3.7 mg/dL, and triglycerides −2.2 mg/dL. Stronger effects were observed for ≥60 g nuts/d.	Del Gobbo [28]
Review of 10 trials, n = 374	37 to 128 g/d	8 to 24 weeks	nut consumption significantly improved flow mediated dilation	Xiao [34]
Review of meta-analyses of prospective studies	Varied	Varied	↓19–20% overall mortality ↓20–34% CHD incidence ↓27–30% CHD mortality ↓19% all CVD incidence ↓25% all CVD mortality ↓10–11% stroke incidence ↓18% stroke mortality	Kim [35]
Meta-analysis of prospective studies	Results per 28 g/d	Varied	↓15% total cancer mortality ↓39% diabetes mortality ↓52% respiratory disease mortality ↓75% infectious disease mortality	Aune [36]
Meta-analysis, 36 studies, n = 30,708 Prospective and case–control studies	Varied	Varied	↓15% total cancer mortality ↓24% colorectal, ↓42% endometrial, ↓32 pancreatic	Wu [37]
Review and meta-analysis, n = 819,851	Highest vs. lowest intake compared	Varied	↓14% cancer risk ↓13% cancer mortality	Naghshi [38]
Golestan Cohort Study, Iran, n = 50,045	3 serving/ wk. vs. none	7 years	↓29% all-cause mortality, nut consumption not associated with healthy lifestyle	Eslamparast [39]
Adventist Health Study, n = 31,208	4x/wk. vs. < 1x/wk	6 years	↓48% CHD mortality, ↓55% definite non-fatal CHD events	Fraser [41]
Adventist Health Study 2, n = 81,337		Median 9.9 years	↓40% risk of CVD death; 3-fold lower for age 25–44	Tharrey [40]

CVD = cardiovascular disease, CHD = coronary heart disease.

Table 5.
Summary of health benefits of nuts and seeds.

cancer death. Optimal results will be realized by optimizing all aspects of dietary and lifestyle choices, but the inclusion of a serving of nuts per day appears to be a wise choice.

4. The safety of nuts and seeds when dealing with cancer

There is one remaining issue to address here. The evidence above indicates that nuts help prevent some cancers, but what is the role of nuts and seeds after diagnosis, or during treatment or remission of cancer?

A more fundamental issue is whether dietary fats cause growth of tumors.

It is well accepted that sugar feeds cancer directly. The PET scan is done on this principle. A sugar molecule with a radiolabeled tracer on it, typically ^{18}F-fluorodeoxyglucose, is injected into a person. Whatever part of the body is metabolizing sugar the fastest is the biggest tumor. Tumors metabolize sugar at an accelerated rate compared to the rest of the body.

Protein may also be a factor in tumor growth. Tumor cells can grow on the amino acid glutamine nearly as well as with glucose as an energy source, especially under low oxygen conditions [42–44]. The TCA cycle that produces energy can run on either glucose or glutamine especially in cancer cells.

Protein can also indirectly feed cancer through hormonal effects. High protein, especially animal protein, raises insulin levels and especially raises IGF-1 levels. IGF-1 is a growth hormone that promotes the growth of all cells. Sufficient levels of IGF-1 prevent frailty but excessive levels have been associated in several studies with higher risk of cancer incidence and death [45].

So, sugar and animal protein both contribute to tumor growth. Does dietary fat also cause tumor growth? It is well known that abdominal fat is a risk factor for cancer. Fat cells in your body produce inflammatory substances. Being overweight or obese is a risk factor for cancer. It has already been established that nuts and seeds do not contribute to obesity in populations that habitually consume them daily.

It turns out that the source of dietary fat makes a difference. It always has, even in the Seven Countries Study on fat and international rates of heart disease deaths [46]. When the analysis is separated into plant fats and animal fats the animal fats appear to be associated with disease, but not plant fats. More recent studies have also found this effect.

In recent analysis of data from two large cohorts of the USA population, the Nurses' Health Study and the Health Professionals Follow-Up Study, the source of MUFAs was separated into plant and animal source. Guasch-Ferré et al. found the MUFAs from plants were associated with lower total mortality and the MUFAs from animals were associated with higher total mortality [47]. Just the opposite effects were seen, depending on the source of the fats. This would indicate that MUFAs from nuts are not in the same category as MUFAs from animal products.

Another recent article also highlighted the difference between MUFAs from plants or animals. The results of analyzing 16 years of follow-up of the NIH-AARP Diet and Health Study with about 520,000 people were that cardiovascular mortality was positively associated with saturated fats, trans fats, arachidonic acid (from animal foods), and animal-sourced MUFAs and was inversely associated with marine omega-3 PUFAs, linoleic acid (omega 6 oil from plants), and plant-sourced MUFAs [48].

So, plant fats are different from animal sourced fats for health outcomes. When looking at the question of whether fat accelerates tumor growth, the source of the fat has to be considered.

A direct answer to our question of the safety of nuts for cancer patients is also available. In a prospective study of colon cancer patients who were enrolled in a randomized adjuvant chemotherapy trial, those that ate two or more servings of tree nuts per week during the 6.5 years of follow-up had a 46 percent improvement in disease-free survival rate and a 53 percent improvement in overall survival [49]. This analysis controlled for other known or suspected risk factors for cancer recurrence, so it appears that the effect is from the nuts themselves. So in this group of cancer patients the ones who ate nuts lived longer without disease and lived longer overall.

Hallelujah Acres and others have advocated the use of flax seeds for cancer patients. The lignans in the fiber of the flax seeds are metabolized into enterodiol and enterolactone, which are well known for reducing cancer risk [50]. Ground flax seeds are considered by many to be a superfood, but while flax seeds are unique, they are a high fat food that has much in common with other nuts and seeds. Sesame seeds also are a precursor source of enterodiol and enterolactone [51]. Other nuts and seeds have phytochemicals in them that appear to be protective to those who eat them as well.

So, the scientific evidence says that nuts and seeds are not only safe, but beneficial in every stage of life, including while battling with cancer. Populations who eat nuts have lower rates of cancer, MUFAs from plants are protective from disease, as opposed to MUFAs from animal sources, there is no clear mechanism for dietary plant fats to accelerate the growth of tumor cells, and a recent clinical trial has shown that intake of nuts by colon cancer patients undergoing chemotherapy had better disease-free survival and overall survival.

5. Conclusion

Let us quickly review the answers to our original queries.

1. Nuts, particularly almonds, and seeds are nutritionally denser than grains, about 43 percent more. Seeds are also about 19 percent more nutritionally dense than dry beans in general.

2. The benefits from one or two ounces of nuts per day are substantial—20% reduction in all-cause mortality, 30% reduction in death by heart disease, 18% reduction in stroke death, 39% reduction in type 2 diabetes death and a 13–15% reduction in cancer death.

3. Nuts are safe to eat when dealing with cancer. Populations who eat nuts have lower rates of cancer and a recent clinical trial has shown that intake of nuts by colon cancer patients undergoing chemotherapy had better disease-free survival and overall survival.

4. The health benefits of nuts and seeds are clear. Nuts and seeds can be easily integrated into any diet. Plant-based diets are improved with nuts and seeds and omnivorous diets, or even low-carbohydrate diets can be improved by including nuts and seeds. The evidence is sufficient and conclusive. Nuts and seeds are beneficial foods.

Acknowledgements

A special thanks to Olin Idol for constructive conversations and suggestions for improving this manuscript.

Conflict of interest

The author declares no conflict of interest.

Author details

Michael S. Donaldson
Hallelujah Acres, Zillah, USA

*Address all correspondence to: mdonaldson@myhdiet.com

References

[1] Ornish D, Brown SE, Scherwitz LW, Billings JH, Armstrong WT, Ports TA, et al. Can lifestyle changes reverse coronary heart disease? The lifestyle heart trial. Lancet. 1990;**336**(8708): 129-133. DOI: 10.1016/0140-6736(90) 91656-U

[2] Esselstyn CB, Gendy G, Doyle J, Golubic M, Roizen MF. A way to reverse CAD? The Journal of Family Practice. 2014;**63**(7):356-364b

[3] Campbell EK, Fidahusain M, Campbell TM II. Evaluation of an eight-week whole-food plant-based lifestyle modification program. Nutrients. 2019; **11**(9):2068. DOI: 10.3390/nu11092068

[4] Melina V, Craig W, Levin S. Position of the academy of nutrition and dietetics: Vegetarian diets. Journal of the Academy of Nutrition and Dietetics. 2016;**116**(12): 1970-1980. DOI: 10.1016/j.jand.2016.09.025

[5] Fuhrman J, Ferreri D. Fueling the vegetarian (vegan) athlete. Current Sports Medicine Reports. 2010;**9**(4):233-241. DOI: 10.1249/JSR.0b013e3181e93a6f

[6] Mariotti F, Gardner CD. Dietary protein and amino acids in vegetarian diets-a review. Nutrients. 2019;**11**(11): 2661. DOI: 10.3390/nu11112661

[7] Godwin N, Roberts T, Hooshmand S, Kern M, Hong MY. Mixed nuts may promote satiety while maintaining stable blood glucose and insulin in healthy, obese, and overweight adults in a two-arm randomized controlled trial. Journal of Medicinal Food. 2019;**22**(4):427-432. DOI: 10.1089/jmf.2018.0127

[8] Vuksan V, Choleva L, Jovanovski E, Jenkins A, Au-Yeung F, Dias A, et al. Comparison of flax (Linum usitatissimum) and Salba-chia (*Salvia hispanica* L.) seeds on postprandial glycemia and satiety in healthy individuals: A randomized, controlled, crossover study. European Journal of Clinical Nutrition. 2017;**71**(2):234-238. DOI: 10.1038/ejcn.2016.148

[9] Yaacoub R, Saliba R, Nsouli B, Khalaf G, Birlouez-Aragon I. Formation of lipid oxidation and isomerization products during processing of nuts and sesame seeds. Journal of Agricultural and Food Chemistry. 2008;**56**(16): 7082-7090. DOI: 10.1021/jf800808d

[10] Brenna JT, Salem N, Sinclair AJ, Cunnane SC. alpha-Linolenic acid supplementation and conversion to n-3 long-chain polyunsaturated fatty acids in humans. Prostaglandins, Leukotrienes, and Essential Fatty Acids. 2009;**80**(2–3): 85-91. DOI: 10.1016/j.plefa.2009.01.004

[11] Sala-Vila A, Fleming J, Kris-Etherton P, Ros E. Impact of α-linolenic acid, the vegetable ω-3 fatty acid, on cardiovascular disease and cognition. Advances in Nutrition (Bethesda, Md.). 2022;**13**(5):1584-1602. DOI: 10.1093/advances/nmac016

[12] Sacks FM, Lichtenstein AH, Wu JHY, Appel LJ, Creager MA, Kris-Etherton PM, et al. Dietary fats and cardiovascular disease: A presidential advisory from the American heart association. Circulation. 2017;**16**(3): e1-e23. DOI: 10.1161/CIR.00000000000 00510

[13] Jung H, Chen CYO, Blumberg JB, Kwak HK. The effect of almonds on vitamin E status and cardiovascular risk factors in Korean adults: A randomized clinical trial. European Journal of Nutrition. 2018;**57**(6):2069-2079. DOI: 10.1007/s00394-017-1480-5

[14] USDA. Usual nutrient intake from food and beverages, by gender and age. In: What We Eat in America, NHANES 2013–2016. Beltsville, MD: Agricultural Research Service; 2019

[15] Barbagallo M, Veronese N, Dominguez LJ. Magnesium in aging, health and diseases. Nutrients. 2021; **13**(2):463. DOI: 10.3390/nu13020463

[16] The Magpie Trial Collaborative Group. Do women with pre-eclampsia, and their babies, benefit from magnesium sulphate? The Magpie trial: A randomised placebo-controlled trial. The Lancet. 2002;**359**(9321):1877-1890

[17] Zhang Z, Cogswell ME, Gillespie C, Fang J, Loustalot F, Dai S, et al. Association between usual sodium and potassium intake and blood pressure and hypertension among U.S. adults: NHANES 2005–2010. PLoS One. 2013; **8**(10):e75289. DOI: 10.1371/journal.pone.0075289

[18] Macdonald HM, New SA, Fraser WD, Campbell MK, Reid DM. Low dietary potassium intakes and high dietary estimates of net endogenous acid production are associated with low bone mineral density in premenopausal women and increased markers of bone resorption in postmenopausal women. The American Journal of Clinical Nutrition. 2005;**81**(4):923-933

[19] Narasaki Y, You AS, Malik S, Moore LW, Bross R, Cervantes MK, et al. Dietary potassium intake, kidney function, and survival in a nationally representative cohort. The American Journal of Clinical Nutrition. 2022;**116**(4):1123-1134. DOI: 10.1093/ajcn/nqac215

[20] Zhang J, Saad R, Taylor EW, Rayman MP. Selenium and selenoproteins in viral infection with potential relevance to COVID-19. Redox Biology. 2020;**37**:101715. DOI: 10.1016/j.redox.2020.101715

[21] Sadeghsoltani F, Mohammadzadeh I, Safari MM, Hassanpour P, Izadpanah M, Qujeq D, et al. Zinc and respiratory viral infections: Important trace element in anti-viral response and immune regulation. Biological Trace Element Research. 2021;**200**:2556-2571. DOI: 10.1007/s12011-021-02859-z

[22] Gao JW, Zhang SL, Hao QY, Huang FF, Liu ZY, Zhang HF, et al. Association of dietary zinc intake with coronary artery calcium progression: The multi-ethnic study of atherosclerosis (MESA). European Journal of Nutrition. 2021;**60**(5):2759-2767. DOI: 10.1007/s00394-020-02452-5

[23] Swaminath S, Um CY, Prizment AE, Lazovich D, Bostick RM. Combined mineral intakes and risk of colorectal cancer in postmenopausal women. Cancer Epidemiology Biomarkers & Prevention. 2019;**28**(2):392-399. DOI: 10.1158/1055-9965.EPI-18-0412

[24] Flores-Mateo G, Rojas-Rueda D, Basora J, Ros E, Salas-Salvadó J. Nut intake and adiposity: Meta-analysis of clinical trials. The American Journal of Clinical Nutrition. 2013;**97**(6):1346-1355. DOI: 10.3945/ajcn.111.031484

[25] Bes-Rastrollo M, Wedick NM, Martinez-Gonzalez MA, Li TY, Sampson L, Hu FB. Prospective study of nut consumption, long-term weight change, and obesity risk in women. The American Journal of Clinical Nutrition. 2009;**89**(6):1913-1919. DOI: 10.3945/ajcn.2008.27276

[26] Freisling H, Noh H, Slimani N, Chajès V, May AM, Peeters PH, et al. Nut intake and 5-year changes in body

weight and obesity risk in adults: Results from the EPIC-PANACEA study. European Journal of Nutrition. 2018; **57**(7):2399-2408. DOI: 10.1007/ s00394-017-1513-0

[27] Tan SY, Mattes RD. Appetitive, dietary and health effects of almonds consumed with meals or as snacks: A randomized, controlled trial. European Journal of Clinical Nutrition. 2013; **67**(11):1205-1214. DOI: 10.1038/ ejcn.2013.184

[28] Del Gobbo LC, Falk MC, Feldman R, Lewis K, Mozaffarian D. Effects of tree nuts on blood lipids, apolipoproteins, and blood pressure: Systematic review, meta-analysis, and dose-response of 61 controlled intervention trials. The American Journal of Clinical Nutrition. 2015;**102**(6):1347-1356. DOI: 10.3945/ ajcn.115.110965

[29] Guasch-Ferré M, Li J, Hu FB, Salas-Salvadó J, Tobias DK. Effects of walnut consumption on blood lipids and other cardiovascular risk factors: An updated meta-analysis and systematic review of controlled trials. The American Journal of Clinical Nutrition. 2018;**108**(1): 174-187. DOI: 10.1093/ajcn/nqy091

[30] Musa-Veloso K, Paulionis L, Poon T, Lee HY. The effects of almond consumption on fasting blood lipid levels: A systematic review and meta-analysis of randomised controlled trials. Journal of Nutritional Science. 2016;**5**: e34. DOI: 10.1017/jns.2016.19

[31] Mohammadifard N, Salehi-Abargouei A, Salas-Salvadó J, Guasch-Ferré M, Humphries K, Sarrafzadegan N. The effect of tree nut, peanut, and soy nut consumption on blood pressure: A systematic review and meta-analysis of randomized controlled clinical trials. The American Journal of Clinical Nutrition. 2015;**101**(5):966-982. DOI: 10.3945/ ajcn.114.091595

[32] Neale EP, Tapsell LC, Guan V, Batterham MJ. The effect of nut consumption on markers of inflammation and endothelial function: A systematic review and meta-analysis of randomised controlled trials. BMJ Open. 2017;**7**(11):e016863. DOI: 10.1136/ bmjopen-2017-016863

[33] Thijssen DHJ, Black MA, Pyke KE, Padilla J, Atkinson G, Harris RA, et al. Assessment of flow-mediated dilation in humans: A methodological and physiological guideline. American Journal of Physiology. Heart and Circulatory Physiology. 2011;**300**(1):H2-H12. DOI: 10.1152/ajpheart.00471.2010

[34] Xiao Y, Huang W, Peng C, Zhang J, Wong C, Kim JH, et al. Effect of nut consumption on vascular endothelial function: A systematic review and meta-analysis of randomized controlled trials. Clinical Nutrition. 2018;**37**(3):831-839. DOI: 10.1016/j.clnu.2017.04.011

[35] Kim Y, Keogh J, Clifton PM. Nuts and cardio-metabolic disease: A review of meta-analyses. Nutrients. 2018; **10**(12):1935. DOI: 10.3390/nu10121935

[36] Aune D, Keum N, Giovannucci E, Fadnes LT, Boffetta P, Greenwood DC, et al. Nut consumption and risk of cardiovascular disease, total cancer, all-cause and cause-specific mortality: A systematic review and dose-response meta-analysis of prospective studies. BMC Medicine. 2016;**14**(1):207. DOI: 10.1186/s12916-016-0730-3

[37] Wu L, Wang Z, Zhu J, Murad AL, Prokop LJ, Murad MH. Nut consumption and risk of cancer and type 2 diabetes: A systematic review and meta-analysis. Nutrition Reviews. 2015;**73**(7):409-425. DOI: 10.1093/nutrit/nuv006

[38] Naghshi S, Sadeghian M, Nasiri M, Mobarak S, Asadi M, Sadeghi O. Association of total nut, tree nut, peanut, and peanut butter consumption with cancer incidence and mortality: A comprehensive systematic review and dose-response meta-analysis of observational studies. Advances in Nutrition (Bethesda, Md.). 2021;**12**(3): 793-808. DOI: 10.1093/advances/nmaa152

[39] Eslamparast T, Sharafkhah M, Poustchi H, Hashemian M, Dawsey SM, Freedman ND, et al. Nut consumption and total and cause-specific mortality: Results from the Golestan cohort study. International Journal of Epidemiology. 2017;**46**(1):75-85. DOI: 10.1093/ije/dyv365

[40] Tharrey M, Mariotti F, Mashchak A, Barbillon P, Delattre M, Fraser GE. Patterns of plant and animal protein intake are strongly associated with cardiovascular mortality: The adventist health study-2 cohort. International Journal of Epidemiology. 2018;**47**(5): 1603-1612. DOI: 10.1093/ije/dyy030

[41] Fraser GE, Sabate J, Beeson WL, Strahan TM. A possible protective effect of nut consumption on risk of coronary heart disease: The adventist health study. Archives of Internal Medicine. 1992; **152**(7):1416-1424. DOI: 10.1001/archinte.1992.00400190054010

[42] Souba W. Glutamine and cancer. Annals of Surgery. 1993 Dec;**218**:6. DOI: 10.1097/00000658-199312000-00004

[43] Li T, Copeland C, Le A. Glutamine metabolism in cancer. Advances in Experimental Medicine and Biology. 2021;**1311**. DOI: 10.1007/978-3-030-65768-0_2

[44] Corbet C, Feron O. Cancer cell metabolism and mitochondria: Nutrient plasticity for TCA cycle fueling. Biochimica Et Biophysica Acta. Reviews on Cancer. 2017;**1868**(1):7-15. DOI: 10.1016/j.bbcan.2017.01.002

[45] Levine ME, Suarez JA, Brandhorst S, Balasubramanian P, Cheng CW, Madia F, et al. Low protein intake is associated with a major reduction in IGF-1, cancer, and overall mortality in the 65 and younger but not older population. Cell Metabolism. 2014;**19**(3): 407-417. DOI: 10.1016/j.cmet.2014.02.006

[46] Menotti A, Kromhout D, Blackburn H, Fidanza F, Buzina R, Nissinen A. Food intake patterns and 25-year mortality from coronary heart disease: Cross-cultural correlations in the seven countries study. The seven countries study research group. European Journal of Epidemiology. 1999; **15**(6):507-515. DOI: 10.1023/a:1007529206050

[47] Guasch-Ferre M, Zong G, Willett WC, Zock P, Wanders AJ, Hu FB, et al. Associations of monounsaturated fatty acids from plant and animal sources with total and cause-specific mortality in two us prospective cohort studies. Circulation Research. 2019;**124**(8):1266-1275. DOI: 10.1161/CIRCRESAHA.118.313996

[48] Zhuang P, Zhang Y, He W, Chen X, Chen J, He L, et al. Dietary fats in relation to total and cause-specific mortality in a prospective cohort of 521,120 individuals with 16 years of follow-up. Circulation Research. 2019; **124**:757-768. DOI: 10.1161/CIRCRESAHA.118.314038

[49] Fadelu T, Zhang S, Niedzwiecki D, Ye X, Saltz LB, Mayer RJ, et al. Nut consumption and survival in patients with stage III colon cancer: Results from

CALGB 89803 (Alliance). Journal of Clinical Oncology. 2018;**36**(11): 1112-1120. DOI: 10.1200/JCO.2017.75.5413

[50] Mason JK, Thompson LU. Flaxseed and its lignan and oil components: Can they play a role in reducing the risk of and improving the treatment of breast cancer? Applied Physiology, Nutrition, and Metabolism. 2014;**39**(6):663-678. DOI: 10.1139/apnm-2013-0420

[51] Coulman KD, Liu Z, Hum WQ, Michaelides J, Thompson LU. Whole sesame seed is as rich a source of mammalian lignan precursors as whole flaxseed. Nutrition and Cancer. 2005; **52**(2):156-165. DOI: 10.1207/s15327914nc5202_6

Chapter 2

African *Moringa stenopetala* Plant: An Emerging Source of Novel Ingredients for Plant-Based Foods

Anteneh T. Tefera, Debebe Worku Dadi, Alemayehu Getahun, Asaminew Abiyu, Alphonsus Utioh, Diriba Muleta, Rotimi E. Aluko and Mulualem T. Kassa

Abstract

Moringa stenopetala is a multi-purpose tropical plant native to East Africa. The plant is exceptionally rich in nutrients and health-promoting bioactive compounds. It is among the top plants that could potentially feed the world and alleviate nutritional deficiencies. *Moringa stenopetala* is a versatile plant because its various parts, including leaves, seeds, flowers, pods, bark, and roots are useful to humans. Especially, the leaves and seeds are high in protein with all the essential amino acids. Based on the FAO database, *M. stenopetala* seed protein with its essential amino acid content stands highest among all commercial plant protein sources. Though it is a high-value plant and extensively used for food and traditional medicine by the local people in its native place, it is underutilized elsewhere. This chapter reviews recent research efforts that aim to unlock the potential of the plant as a source of ingredients for food, cosmetic and nutraceutical industries.

Keywords: bioactive compounds, *Moringa stenopetala*, oil, plant-based food, protein

1. Introduction

The growing awareness of the effects of food on human health and the environment has warranted a need to look for alternative food sources. This has promoted a steady increase in demand for plant-based diets [1], which can be attributed to increasing vegan, vegetarian, and flexitarian populations as well as increasing intolerance to animal proteins. Ethical concerns about animal abuse, the nutritional benefits of plant-based diets and the ever-increasing investments in the plant protein sector are all factors contributing to the growth of plant-based foods [2, 3].

The plant-based food market is expected to grow at a compound annual growth rate (CAGR) of 12.4% in 2022 to reach $95.52 billion by 2029 [2]. The growth rate for the U.S. plant-based food market was more than doubled in 2020 as sales surged 27% to $7 billion, according to the Plant Based Foods Association (PBFA) and Good Food Institute (GFI). To meet the increasing demand, there is a need to adopt climate-resilient food production system with higher yields of improved functional food ingredients. The versatile tropical plant species Moringa with uses for its various parts, particularly the leaves and seeds, holds immense potential for use as ingredients in plant-based food and therapeutic applications.

Moringa belongs to the monogeneric Moringaceae family [4]. The genus consists of about 14 species, including the well-known species, *Moringa oleifera*, which is native to the Indian sub-continent, and *Moringa stenopetala*, also known as African Moringa, which is endemic to East Africa [5]. The leaves and green pods of Moringa are rich in both macro and micro-nutrients and are eaten as a staple vegetable, especially in the Indian sub-continent and Africa [6].

Moringa is one of the world's most useful tropical trees and often nick-named a 'multi-purpose tree' [7, 8]. It is a resilient and highly drought-tolerant tree growing on marginalized land and almost all parts of the plant are useful [9]. The leaves, seeds, pods, flowers, and roots are excellent sources of nutrients and bioactive compounds [10, 11], especially dietary fiber, proteins, minerals, vitamins, and phytochemicals that offer great nutritional and therapeutic benefits [5, 12–14].

Moringa is listed among the top plants that could help feed the world and alleviate nutritional deficiencies and is often considered as a superfood [7, 8]. It holds much promise to serve as a source of valuable bioactive compounds for food, pharmaceutical and cosmetic applications [5]. Moringa seed hulls (often considered a waste) are used to develop high performance carbonaceous adsorbents and biological coagulants for water and wastewater treatment and removal of hazardous contaminants, which enhances environmental health [15–17].

Unlike *M. oleifera* for which there are robust scientific studies on its chemistry, food, and therapeutic uses [12, 13], only a few similar scientific studies have been conducted on *M. stenopetala* [18].

M. stenopetala is used as a staple food and traditional medicine by the local people in its native place in East Africa. It grows on the homesteads of small-holder farmers and is tightly linked to the livelihood of local communities in the region (**Figure 1**). The plant is exceptionally rich in nutrients and health-boosting bioactive compounds and could potentially alleviate nutritional deficiencies. The leaves and seeds are high in protein content and contain all the essential amino acids. Recent studies in Canada revealed that *M. stenopetala* seed protein with its essential amino acid content is the highest among all the commercial plant protein sources based on the FAO database (personal communication).

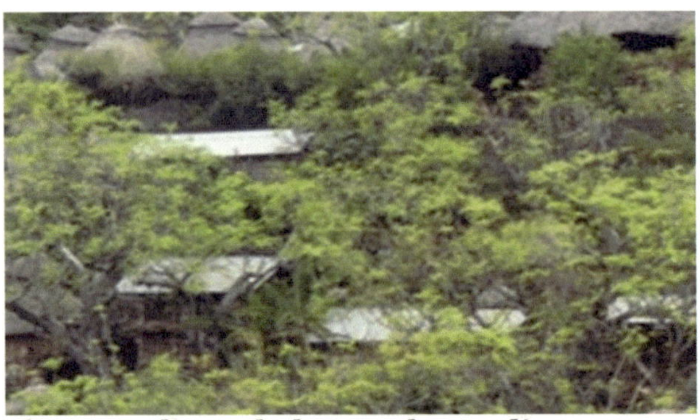

Photo credit: Debebe Worku Dadi

Figure 1.
Moringa stenopetala *in Konso, Southern Ethiopia.*

Though the plant holds much promise as a source of ingredients for nutrient-and mineral-rich plant-based diets, it is less known to the outside world and rarely utilized in food product formulations. Thus, this chapter reviews recent research interests that aim to uncover potential uses of *M. stenopetala* ingredients for plant-based food and therapeutic applications.

2. Origin, ecology, and production of *M. stenopetala*

M. stenopetala is native to east Africa, with diversity spanning Ethiopia, Kenya, and Central Somalia [19]. In Ethiopia, the distribution of the species is mostly concentrated in specific zones in the south [20–23]. The presence of *M. stenopetala* has also been reported in the northern part of the country, specifically in Alamata district of southern Tigray, where it is promoted as an agroforestry tree species [24].

M. stenopetala grows in Ethiopia from 390 to 2200 meters above sea level (mas) in the southern Rift Valley, including the arid and semi-arid regions between 1000 and 1800 mas [23, 25]. *M. stenopetala* grows well in areas receiving annual rainfall and temperature that ranges from 250 to 1500 mm and 25°C to 35°C, respectively. According to a summary of the national herbarium's vouchers, the habitat where the genus occurs in Ethiopia consists of rocky riverbanks, dry scrub land, Acacia-Commiphora woodland, watercourses with some evergreens, open Acacia Commiphora bush land on gray alluvial soil, and cultivated lands in and around villages.

M. stenopetala is intercropped with food crops in moderately dry regions of southern Ethiopia and used as a farm tree (home gardens) to support the livelihoods of the high population present in the region. It is among the most useful trees planted and managed by rural people in the dry areas of Ethiopia [7, 26]. With proper agronomic practices, *M. stenopetala* has the potential for large-scale commercial farming. It was reported that a single tree of *M. stenopetala* could support a large family for several years [21, 27]. Thus, *M. stenopetala* is a promising plant to adopt for a climate-resilient food production system that could have a significant impact on alleviating food insecurity and serve as a source of ingredients in food and therapeutic applications.

3. Nutrient and bioactive composition of various parts of *M. stenopetala*

The nutrient, bioactive compounds, vitamin, and mineral composition of various parts of the plant, particularly the leaves and seeds, are presented in this section. The trending potential of the use of *M. stenopetala* ingredients in plant-food formulations is also highlighted. The nutritional and bioactive composition of *M. stenopetala* is presented and compared with that of *M. oleifera*, for which a wealth of information on its chemistry, nutrient and bioactive profiles and therapeutic potential is available [12, 13].

Moringa leaves, seeds, flowers, roots, and green pods are rich in macro and micronutrients. The leaves of *M. stenopetala* are popular as a staple vegetable in eastern Africa as is *M. oleifera* in the Indian subcontinent [21, 28, 29]. Dried Moringa leaf powder that is kept under dark conditions preserves the nutritional potency of the leaves for a long period of time [30, 31]. Dried leaves are utilized for the preparation of Moringa herbal tea and other non-alcoholic beverages that have significant health benefits [18].

3.1 Dietary composition of the leaf

Findings from various studies revealed that *M. stenopetala* and *M. oleifera* are rich in nutrients, minerals, vitamins, and bioactive compounds [32]. *M. stenopetala* dried leaf has a high protein content of about 28% (**Figure 2**). The protein from the leaves of *M. stenopetala* is complete and contains all the essential amino acids at levels equal to or higher than those found in soybean seeds [32, 33]. Similarly, recent research conducted in Canada found that *M. stenopetala* leaf has high protein content and contains all the essential amino acids (personal communication).

M. stenopetala leaf contains 28 and 160 mg/100 g of vitamin C and beta carotene, respectively [21]. Some studies have also reported the presence of other vitamins in higher amounts [21, 32]. Among many green leafy vegetables, Moringa was found to be a rich source of ß-carotene (vitamin A) and other micronutrients [34].

Leaf extracts of *M. stenopetala* have good amounts of phenolic and flavonoid compounds that have high antioxidant activities [35, 36]. Habtemariam and Varghese [18] have also reported the presence of a high amount of rutin, a bioflavonoid antioxidant that could be extracted from *M. stenopetala*'s dried leaves.

Previously published papers demonstrated that the minerals found in Moringa leaves are diverse and abundant. *M. stenopetala* leaves had 3363 mg/100 g of potassium, which was 3.96 times higher than in banana fruit (933 mg/100 g) [37]. Banana fruit is one of the foods recommended as a source of potassium and calcium [38]. *M. stenopetala* dried leaf is rich in calcium, potassium, magnesium, iron, phosphorus, and zinc but characterized by its low content of sodium [37]. *M. stenopetala* is nutrient-rich but low-calorie food and is an ideal part of a diet designed for body weight management.

3.2 Composition of *M. stenopetala* seed

Different research results have reported protein (28–43%) and oil (33–41%) levels from *M. stenopetala* seeds. *M. stenopetala* seeds are a great source of protein, high-quality edible oil, and numerous other beneficial compounds [12]. Studies have shown high protein content and considerable levels of essential amino acids in

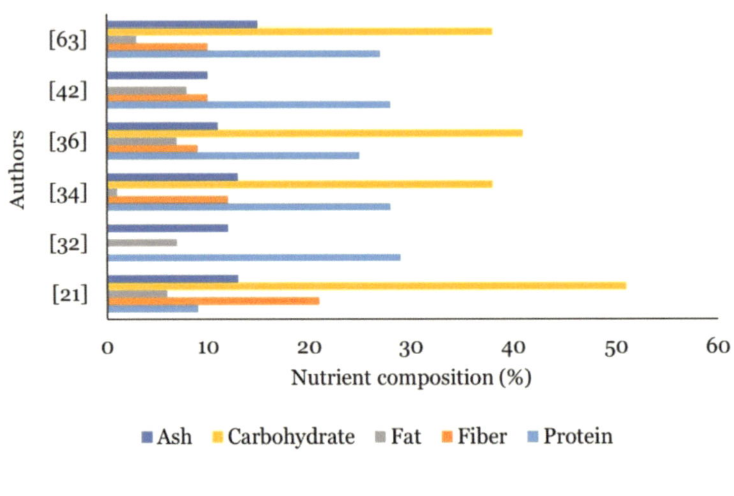

Figure 2.
Nutrient composition (%) of Moringa stenopetala *dried leaves (adapted from authors indicated on the above chart).*

Moringa seeds [12]. Results of different studies on the amino acids exhibited high qualities of the seed protein [39, 40]. Various studies have shown that the protein from Moringa seeds contains all nine essential amino acids, making it one of the best sources of plant-based proteins [12, 41, 42].

The amino acid composition of Moringa seed was compared to the hen's egg used as the reference by the FAO [43], and assessed the protein quality using the individual amino acid score. The results of this study showed that Moringa seed proteins have higher amounts of total amino acids and fewer amounts of total essential amino acids than hen's egg protein, revealing the potential use of Moringa seed protein in food applications.

According to the report, 45% of *M. stenopetala* seed is oil, with 78% of the fatty acid composition being monounsaturated (of which 76% is oleic) and 22% is saturated fatty acids [22]. *M. stenopetala* seed oil has an average value of oil density (0.919 kg/cm^3), specific gravity (0.918 g/cm^3), peroxide value (11.52 millieq O_2/kg), viscosity (19 mPa.s), acid value (3.74 mg KOH/g) and ester value (177.2 mg KOH/g) [44, 45]. According to Vaknin and Mishal [46], the saturated fatty acids present in Moringa oil include palmitic acid, stearic acid, arachidic acid, and behenic acid. The unique fatty acid and bioactive components, combined with distinct physiochemical properties, make *M. stenopetala* oil an ideal ingredient for food, pharmaceutical, cosmeceutical, and therapeutic applications [43, 47].

3.3 Pods and other parts

Moringa stenopetala's flower, pod, and roots have received much less attention and are less known than the leaves and seeds. The protein, fiber, and ash contents of the pods of *M. stenopetala* and *M. oleifera* were 18 and 17%, 37 and 36%, and 12 and 10%, respectively [48]. The authors have also reported the mineral contents of pods of *M. stenopetala* and *M. oleifera* (**Figure 3**) with the further remark that the flowers, pods, and roots of Moringa contain appreciable concentrations of minerals and nutrients. Therefore, *M. stenopetala* enhances dietary diversification and thus has a significant impact on mitigating hunger in developing countries.

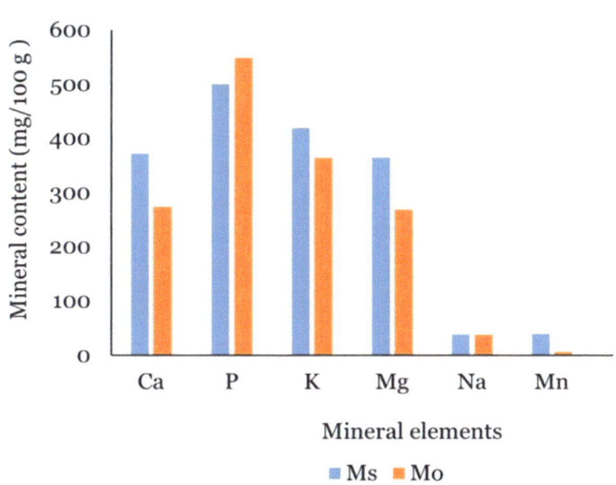

Figure 3.
Mineral contents of pods of M. stenopetala *(Ms) and* M. oleifera *(Mo) [48].*

4. Health benefits of *Moringa stenopetala* diet

The health benefits of *M. oleifera* are well documented in recent research reports [12, 13]. Though we have a dearth of information, some studies have also shown the nutritional and health benefits of *M. stenopetala*. Different parts of the plant are traditionally used to treat hypertension, diabetes, malaria, common cold, asthma, wounds, retained placenta, and stomach-ache [49, 50]. The leaf extracts of *M. stenopetala* have shown antihypertensive effects and antidiabetic activity [51, 52]. Furthermore, hepato- and kidney protective effects of Moringa leaf extracts were also reported [53]. This might be due to the presence of protective action against lipid peroxidation and reactive oxygen species of the plant's extract, which can be attributed to the presence of phenolic and flavonoid compounds [18, 54]. *M. stenopetala* leaf extract also has a high content of rutin, a powerful bioflavonoid [18]. These compounds exhibit higher antioxidant activity and are claimed to be responsible for several beneficial biological activities.

Diabetes mellitus is a complex metabolic disease that is a major global public health concern. Diabetes is increasing at an alarming rate all over the world and its prevention will necessitate measures to promote a healthy dietary pattern. Studies revealed that *M. stenopetala* leaf extract has the potential to reduce blood glucose levels effectively [55, 56]. Serum glucose level was also decreased significantly after 6 weeks of treatment of mice with *M. stenopetala* leaf extract [57]. In addition, microencapsulated products developed from *M. stenopetala* leaf extracts have shown a significant effect on diabetes [52]. The leaf of *M. stenopetala* also has a high dietary fiber [21], which may help in the prevention and management of diabetes. Furthermore, the phenolic compounds, vitamin E and tannins, present in *M. stenopetala*, can also help to reduce the risk of diabetes by managing blood glucose levels.

M. stenopetala leaf extract showed an antihypertensive activity as it was found from the result of vasodilator and urinary excretion increment [52]. The decreased blood pressure, extracellular fluid volume, and cardiac output occurred due to diuretics, which increase the urinary sodium excretion, thereby reducing the plasma volume that controls hypertension [58]. *M. stenopetala* leaf extract has shown significant diuretic activity [51, 52], consequently it has the potential to act as an antihypertensive agent.

The relaxation of the smooth muscle of blood vessels (vasodilation) favors normal blood pressure. However, if this blood vessel is contracted, relaxation is required using nitric oxide [59]. It was found that *M. stenopetala* leaf extract has a high relaxation (99.13%) against potassium chloride induced contraction of the guinea pig thoracic aorta at a concentration of 40 mg/mL [52]. Oral administration of the aqueous extract of *M. stenopetala* leaves led to significant reductions in systolic blood pressure, diastolic blood pressure and mean arterial blood pressure [16].

It is claimed that *M. stenopetala* has anti-carcinogenic activities due to the presence of glucosinolate compounds [60]. In addition, *M. stenopetala* leaf extract contains polyphenols and flavonoids that give a synergistic effect to anti-carcinogenic activities [54, 60].

5. Trends of *Moringa stenopetala* use in food and nutraceutical applications

M. stenopetala is emerging as a trending source of novel ingredients in the food, pharmaceutical and skin care industries. The dried leaves are used to formulate health-boosting herbal tea, the dried leaf powder is a source of nutrient-dense

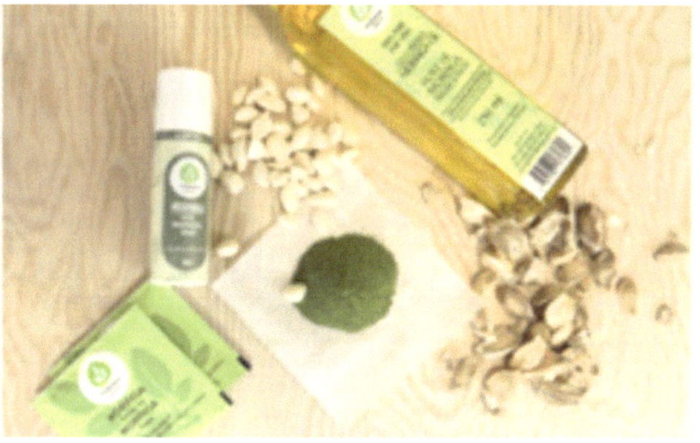

Figure 4.
Commercialized herbal tea, leaf protein powder, seed oil and moisturizing facial cream developed from M. stenopetala *leaves and seeds through research and development project in Canada (Photo credit: BioTEI Inc.).*

ingredient for food applications, and the seed oil is used by the food and skin care industries (**Figure 4**). After the oil is extracted from the seed, it leaves a protein-rich press cake as a secondary extraction product.

The seeds of *M. stenopetala* are good sources of edible oil and flocculent agents for water purification as well as biofuel [49]. It was found that the protein content of *M. stenopetala* seed was higher than the protein content of other oilseeds and pulses [45]. This shows that *M. stenopetala* seeds can be utilized as a potential protein source to combat malnutrition in developing countries and as an ingredient for food applications in general. *M. stenopetala* seed oil yield reaches about 44% [61], which can be considered as a major source of oil that could be used for cooking, salad dressing, and cosmetics applications. Moringa oil is also known as ben oil and has been reported to have physical and chemical properties comparable to olive oil with a high concentration of tocopherols and oleic fatty acid [61]. Thus, this oil has better oxidative stability, which can be used in the food industry for longer storage and high-temperature frying. Furthermore, *M. stenopetala* seed oil has excellent absorbing properties on the skin which makes it a vital ingredient for the cosmetic industry. Moringa oil also has anti-aging properties due to its key bio-agents that could maintain moisture and promote the mechanical elasticity and flexibility of the skin [62]. These findings indicate that *M. stenopetala* seed oil is an ideal candidate for the pharmaceutical and cosmetics industries manifesting its untapped multifaceted business potential.

5.1 Food fortification

M. stenopetala enhances dietary diversification and thus has a significant impact on mitigating hunger in developing countries. The leaves are consumed as cabbage and the dried powder is used as a dietary supplement for proteins, calcium, iron, phosphorous as well as vitamins [63, 64]. The essential amino acids concentration of *M. stenopetala* leaves is comparable with that of defatted soybean seed meal [63]. The author has also reported the metabolizable energy, organic matter digestibility, and short chain fatty acids contents. *M. stenopetala* is a rich source of micronutrients that are commonly deficient in cereal-based diets. The concentrations of essential minerals in *M. stenopetala* leaf are very high [7], indicating its superiority to other staple foods grown in Ethiopia (**Table 1**). Moreover, cooking improved the digestibility of protein

Crop	Concentration (mg/kg dw)					
	Ca	Cu	Fe	Mg	Se	Zn
M. stenopetala leaves	19,400	4.71	117	6070	1.12	21.0
Maize grain	55.1	0.943	28.2	918	0.182	20.4
Enset	2190	1.3	71.3	260	0.060	34.2
Sorghum grain	176	1.74	51.5	1350	0.097	16.1
Beans	1500	9.41	88.5	88.5	0.150	24.9

Data adapted from Kumssa et al. [7].

Table 1.
Medial elemental concentrations in M. stenopetala *leaves and other food sources grown in Ethiopia.*

by 20.7 and 7.8% in leaves and pods, respectively; the same trend was observed for the total carbohydrates [64]. These authors have also confirmed the importance of cooking the leaves and pods of *M. stenopetala* for the reduction of tannins (a known anti-nutritional factor) by 27 and 45%, respectively.

The essential amino acids concentration of *M. stenopetala* leaves is comparable with soybean seed meal content [63]. The author has also reported the metabolizable energy, organic matter digestibility, and short-chain fatty acids contents. The leaves of *M. stenopetala* leaves have also relatively high phenolic and flavonoid compounds [18] indicating their antioxidant properties with a health-promoting effect on consumers [54]. Plant-derived bioactive components such as phenolic compounds inhibit the formation of free radicals, thereby preventing the formation of hydroperoxides. However, these bioactive components are lost during food processing using the conventional thermal approach. As a result, fortification is necessary to restore these bioactive components to the final food products, this makes Moringa an incredible ingredient in food fortification.

5.2 Functional and nutraceutical applications

The presence of phenolic and flavonoid compounds helps to prevent oxidative damage. Currently, synthetic antioxidants are reported to be associated with carcinogenic effects; as a result, consumers' interest in natural antioxidant sources is increasing. Nutraceutical, functional foods and pharmaceutical product development have created opportunities for these emerging ingredients derived from Moringa. Functional and nutraceutical products development from *M. stenopetala* extract is a promising strategy to maximize the utilization and industrialization of this underutilized but highly versatile plant. Due to its richness in proteins [63], β-carotene, other bioactive compounds, and antioxidant properties [54] and a high selenium concentration, this plant has untapped potential in human health enhancement [7]. Hence, *M. stenopetala* has the potential to be used as a key ingredient in functional foods and nutraceutical product development.

Environmental variables, storage conditions, and thermal processing, all contribute to the easy degradation of nutritional and bioactive components in *M. stenopetala*. Therefore, it is important to find alternative methods to maintain and improve the stability of these compounds. Product development from *M. stenopetala* is also important to improve the storage stability of the harvested plant parts. Spray-drying microencapsulation of *M. stenopetala* leaf extract using a mixture of maltodextrin and pectin as a coating material is more efficient for the food and pharmaceutical industries than other processes [65]. A microencapsulated product developed from *M. stenopetala* leaf extract showed significant antidiabetic and antihypertensive effects. According to the findings, the percentage of urinary excretion was increased with the increment of the dose of the microencapsulated bioactive product developed from *M. stenopetala* leaf extract [52]. This shows that microencapsulated products have significant diuretic activity. Thus, this microencapsulated product may be used to minimize the abnormal accumulation of fluid in the human/animal body which in turn helps to manage hypertension.

5.3 Antimicrobial properties

Endemic plants, like *M. stenopetala*, are good sources of new antimicrobial compounds that might be effective against microorganisms resistant to commonly prescribed antimicrobials. The leaves/seeds extract from *M. stenopetala* have shown antimicrobial properties. According to Mekonnen and Dräger [60], *M. stenopetala* seed oil extract inhibited the growth of some pathogenic microorganisms such as *Staphylococcus aureus*, *Salmonella typhi*, *Shigella* spp. and *Candida albicans.* Similarly, leaf extracts of *M. stenopetala* using a mixture of methanol and chloroform have significant inhibitory activity against *Klebsiella pneumoniae* and *Bacillus cereus* [66]. Thus, it is important to develop antimicrobial products from *M. stenopetala* as an alternative bio-preservative to improve the shelf stability of some perishable food products.

5.4 Other industrial applications of *Moringa stenopetala* by-products

The seed husk and defatted seed press cake of *M. stenopetala* could be used to develop valuable bio-products (e.g., activated carbons and biological coagulants) that could be utilized in water and wastewater treatment applications that considerably promote a circular economy to enhance environmentally safe clean technology.

6. Conclusion

The African endemic Moringa tree, *M. stenopetala* is well regarded as a beneficial botanical with exceptionally high nutritional and health benefits to humans and thus nicknamed 'the multipurpose tree'. It is highly drought-tolerant and suitable for climate-resilient sustainable food production. Almost all parts of the plant (leaves, flowers, pods, seeds and hulls) have uses in the food, cosmetic and pharmaceutical industries due to their high contents of nutritional and essential bioactive components. Moringa seed oil has a good fatty acid profile suitable for food and cosmetic applications while the press cake (by-product of oil extraction) is rich in protein with good amino acid profile, and dietary fiber, making it a good raw material for protein extraction for the plant-based food industry. The leaves are dried to produce herbal tea, but they can also be ground into nutrient-dense ingredients for the development and fortification of various food products including smoothies, bars, and chips. The hulls can be used to produce activated carbon for water and wastewater treatment. Moringa is a multi-functional plant that is good for human nutrition, environmental health, and plays a pivotal role in economic sustainability of the population. However, more research is required to realize the full potential of *M. stenopetala* through the development of extraction technologies for seed protein and its hydrolysates and fractionated peptides. Research on development of food, cosmetic and nutraceutical products with Moringa ingredients will allow consumers to fully benefit from the nutritional and bioactive components of this African "miracle" tree.

Acknowledgements

The authors thank the National Research Council Canada (NRC)- IRAP program for its support through contribution agreement with BioTEI Inc.

Author details

Anteneh T. Tefera[1,2], Debebe Worku Dadi[3], Alemayehu Getahun[4], Asaminew Abiyu[5], Alphonsus Utioh[6], Diriba Muleta[2], Rotimi E. Aluko[7] and Mulualem T. Kassa[1*]

1 BioTEI Inc., Winnipeg, Manitoba, Canada

2 Institute of Biotechnology, College of Natural Sciences, Addis Ababa University, Ethiopia

3 Department of Food Process Engineering and Postharvest Technology, Institute of Technology, Ambo University, Ethiopia

4 Wachemo University, Hosaena, Ethiopia

5 College of Environmental Science and Engineering, Donghua University, Shanghai, China

6 ACU Food Technology Services Inc., Portage la Prairie, Manitoba, Canada

7 Department of Food and Human Nutritional Sciences, University of Manitoba, Winnipeg, MB, Canada

*Address all correspondence to: mtkassa@bioteinnova.ca

References

[1] Daniel IO, Kassa MT. Advances in food development with plant-based proteins from seed sources. In: Jimenez-Lopez GC, editor. Grain and Seed Proteins Functionality. London: IntechOpen; 2021

[2] Meticulousc MR. Plant based food market worth $95.52 Billion by 2029 [Internet]. 2022. Available from: https://www.meticulousresearch.com/pressrelease/53/plant-based-food-market-2029 [Accessed: February 02, 2023]

[3] Chandra SP, Vianney YM, Christie TL, Wongso M, Widjaja M, Yang DC, et al. Mass production of *Panax ginseng* C.A. Mey. Root cultures in Indonesia. Sarhad Journal of Agriculture. 2006;**37**(1):98-109

[4] Yang RY, Tsou SC, Lee TC, Chang LC, Kuo G, Lai PY. Moringa, a novel plant rich in antioxidants, bioavailable iron, and nutrients. In: Wang M, Sang S, Hwang LC, Ho CT, editors. Herbs: Challenges in Chemistry and Biology. Washington, USA: ACS Publications; 2006

[5] Jahn SAA. The traditional domestication of a multipurpose tree *Moringa stenopetala (Bak. f.)* Cuf. in the Ethiopian Rift Valley. Ambio. 1991;**20**(6):244-247

[6] Seifu E. Actual and potential applications of *Moringa stenopetala*, underutilized indigenous vegetable of Southern Ethiopia: A review. International Journal of Agricultural and Food Research. 2015;**3**(4):8-19

[7] Kumssa DB, Joy EJ, Young SD, Odee DW, Ander EL, Broadely MR. Variation in the mineral element concentration of *Moringa oleifera* Lam. and *M. stenopetala (Bak. f.)* Cuf.: Role in human nutrition. PLoS One. 2017;**12**(4):e0175503. DOI: 10.1371/journal.pone.0175503

[8] Raghavendra H, Kekuda T, Vijayananda B, Duressa D, Solomon T. Nutritive composition and antimicrobial activity of *Moringa stenopetala (Baker f.)* Cufod. Journal of Advances in Medical and Pharmaceutical Sciences. 2016;**10**(3):1-9

[9] Nibret E, Wink M. Trypanocidal and antileukaemic effects of the essential oils of *Hagenia abyssinica, Leonotis ocymifolia, Moringa stenopetala,* and their main individual constituents. Phytomedicine. 2010;**17**(12):911-920

[10] Jain A, Subramanian R, Manohar B, Radha C. Preparation, characterization and functional properties of *Moringa oleifera* seed protein isolate. Journal of Food Science and Technology. 2019;**56**(4):2093-2104

[11] Vats S, Gupta T. Evaluation of bioactive compounds and antioxidant potential of hydroethanolic extract of Moringa oleifera Lam. from Rajasthan, India. Physiology and Molecular Biology of Plants. 2017;**23**(1):239-248

[12] Aderinola TA, Fagbemi TN, Enujiugha VN, Alashi AM, Aluko RE. Amino acid composition and antioxidant properties of *Moringa oleifera* seed protein isolate and enzymatic hydrolysates. Heliyon. 2018;**4**(10):e00877. DOI: 10.1016/j.heliyon.2018.e00877

[13] Aderinola TA, Fagbemi TN, Enujiugha VN, Alashi AM, Aluko RE. *Moringa oleifera* flour protein fractions

as food ingredients with antioxidant properties. SDRP Journal of Food Science and Technology. 2019;**4**(4):720-728

[14] Gopalakrishnan L, Doriya K, Kumar DS. *Moringa oleifera:* A review on nutritive importance and its medicinal application. Food Science and Human Wellness. 2016;**5**(2):49-56

[15] Dondee K, Bootprom P, Saiphet B, Borkaew P, Klubsri C, Somsak V. Antimalarial activities of *Moringa oleifera* leaf extract against *Plasmodium berghei* ANKA infection in ICR mice. International Journal of Innovative Research in Medical Science. 2016;**1**(5):194-201

[16] Mengistu M, Abebe Y, Mekonnen Y, Tolessa T. *In vivo* and *in vitro* hypotensive effect of aqueous extract of *Moringa stenopetala*. African Health Sciences. 2013;**12**(4):545-551

[17] Chumark P, Khunawat P, Sanvarinda Y, Phornchirasilp S, Morales NP, Phivthong-Ngam L, et al. The in vitro and ex vivo antioxidant properties, hypolipidaemic and antiatherosclerotic activities of water extract of *Moringa oleifera* Lam. leaves. Journal of Ethnopharmacology. 2008;**116**(3):439-446

[18] Habtemariam S, Varghese GK. Extractability of rutin in herbal tea preparations of *Moringa stenopetala* leaves. Beverages. 2015;**1**(3):169-182

[19] Al-Thobaiti SA, Zeid IA. Medicinal properties of desert date plants *(Balanites aegyptiaca)*: An overview. Global Journal of Pharmacology. 2018;**12**(1):01-12

[20] Lock M, Edwards S, Tadesse M, Demissew S, Hedberg I. Flora of Ethiopia and Eritrea. Volume 2, Part 2. *Magnoliaceae* to *Flacourtiaceae*. Kew Bulletin. 2001;**56**(2):490

[21] Abuye C, Urga K, Knapp H, Selmar D, Omwega A, Imungi J, et al. A compositional study of *Moringa stenopetala* leaves. East African Medical Journal. 2003;**80**(5):247-252

[22] Ejigu A, Asfaw A, Asfaw N, Licence P. *Moringa stenopetala* seed oil as a potential feedstock for biodiesel production in Ethiopia. Green Chemistry. 2010;**12**(2):316-320

[23] Gebregiorgis F, Negesse T, Nurfeta A. Feed intake and utilization in sheep fed graded levels of dried moringa (*Moringa stenopetala*) leaf as a supplement to Rhodes grass hay. Tropical Animal Health Production. 2012;**44**(3):511-517

[24] Abay A, Birhane E, Tadesse T, Hadgu KM. *Moringa stenopetala* tree species improved selected soil properties and socio-economic benefits in tigray, northern Ethiopia. Science, Technology and Arts Research Journal. 2016;**4**(2):68-78

[25] Jiru D, Sonder K, Alemayehu L, Mekonen Y, Anjulo A. Leaf yield and nutritive value of *Moringa stenopetala* and *Moringa oleifera* accessions: Its potential role in food security in constrained dry farming agroforestry system. In: Proceedings of the Moringa and Other Highly Nutritious Plant Resources: Strategies, Standards and Markets for a Better Impact on Nutrition in Africa; 16-18 November 2006. Accra, Ghana; 2006. pp. 1-14

[26] Taye T, Tesfaye Y. Role of *Moringa stenopetala* based agroforestry practice on rural household economy in Offa Woreda, southern Ethiopia. International Journal of Economy, Energy and Environment. 2021;**6**(2):29-34

[27] Yisehak K, Solomon M, Tadelle M. Contribution of Moringa (*Moringa stenopetala, Bac.*), a highly nutritious

vegetable tree, for food security in south Ethiopia: A review. Asian Journal of Applied Science. 2011;**4**(5):477-488

[28] Abdulkadir AR, Hasan MM, Jahan MS. Antimalarial, antioxidant, antimicrobial properties of *Moringa Oliefera* lam*:* A review. Australian Journal of Crop Science. 2018;**12**(6):905-908

[29] Bello OS, Lasisi BM, Adigun OJ, Ephraim V. Scavenging Rhodamine B dye using *Moringa oleifera* seed pod. Chemical Speciation and Bioavailability. 2017;**29**(1):120-134

[30] Arabshahi-D S, Devi DV, Urooj A. Evaluation of antioxidant activity of some plant extracts and their heat, pH and storage stability. Food Chemistry. 2007;**100**(3):1100-1105

[31] Fahey JW. *Moringa oleifera:* A review of the medical evidence for its nutritional, therapeutic, and prophylactic properties. Trees for Life Journal. 2005;**1**(5):1-15

[32] Kim YJ, Kim HS. Screening Moringa species focused on development of locally available sustainable nutritional supplements. Nutrition Research and Practice. 2019;**13**(6):529-534

[33] Melesse A, Tiruneh W, Negesse T. Effects of feeding *Moringa stenopetala* leaf meal on nutrient intake and growth performance of Rhode Island Red chicks under tropical climate. Tropical and Subtropical Agroecosystems. 2011;**14**(2):485-492

[34] Tekle A, Belay A, Kelem K, Yohannes M, Wodajo B, Tesfaye Y. Nutritional profile of *Moringa stenopetala s*pecies samples collected from different places in Ethiopia. European Journal of Nutrition and Food Safety. 2015;**5**(5):1100-1101

[35] Dessalegn E, Rupasinghe HPV. Phenolic compounds and in vitro antioxidant activity of *Moringa stenopetala* grown in South Ethiopia. International Journal of Food Properties. 2021;**24**(1):1681-1692

[36] Befa A, Gebre A, Bekele T. Evaluation of nutritional properties of dried Moringa *(Moringa stenopetala)* leaves and dried Moringa leaves infusion. Medicinal and Aromat Plants. 2020;**9**(6):363. DOI: 10.35248/2167-0412.20.9.363

[37] Gurmessa BK, Geleta GS, Tsadik GG. Comparison of potassium content of *Moringa stenopetala* and banana sold at local market in Jimma town, Oromia, south west Ethiopia. World Journal of Pharmaceutical Research. 2015;**4**(1):1173-1178

[38] Wall MM. Ascorbic acid, vitamin A, and mineral composition of banana (*Musa sp.*) and papaya (*Carica papaya*) *cultivars grown in Hawaii*. Journal of Food Composition and Analysis. 2006;**19**(5):434-445

[39] Kumar M, Selvasekaran P, Kapoor S, Barbhai MD, Lorenzo JM, Saurabh V, et al. *Moringa oleifera* lam. seed proteins: Extraction, preparation of protein hydrolysates, bioactivities, functional food properties, and industrial application. Food Hydrocolloids. 2022;**2022**:131. DOI: 10.1016/j.foodhyd.2022.107791

[40] Mune MA, Nyobe EC, Bassogog CB, Minka SR. A comparison on the nutritional quality of proteins from *Moringa oleifera* leaves and seeds. Cogent Food and Agriculture. 2016;**2**(1):1213618. DOI: 10.1080/23311932.2016.1213618

[41] Ogunsina BS, Radha C, Indrani D. Quality characteristics of bread and cookies enriched with debittered

Moringa oleifera seed flour. International Journal of Food Science and Nutrition. 2011;**62**(2):185-194

[42] Melesse A, Bulang M, Kluth H. Evaluating the nutritive values andin vitrodegradability characteristics of leaves, seeds and seedpods from *Moringa stenopetala*. Journal of the Science of Food and Agriculture. 2009;**89**(2):281-287

[43] Barakat H, Ghazal GA. Physicochemical properties of *Moringa oleifera* seeds and their edible oil cultivated at different regions in Egypt. Food and Nutrition Sciences. 2016;7(6):472-484

[44] Gisila T. Extraction, Kinetics Study and Characterization of *Moringa Stenopetala* Seed Oil. Addis Ababa: School of Chemical and Bio Engineering, Addis Ababa University; 2018

[45] Shumi LD, Bacha EG, Carotenuto G. Studies on modeling and physicochemical properties of oil extracted from *Moringa stenopetala seed*. Advances in Materials Science and Engineering. 2022;**2022**:1-9. DOI: 10.1155/2022/4539533

[46] Vaknin Y, Mishal A. The potential of the tropical "miracle tree" *Moringa oleifera* and its desert relative *Moringa peregrina* as edible seed-oil and protein crops under Mediterranean conditions. Scientia Horticulturae. 2017;**225**:431-437. DOI: 10.1016/j.scienta.2017.07.039

[47] Boukandoul S, Casal S, Zaidi F. The potential of some Moringa species for seed oil production. Agriculture. 2018;**8**(10):150. DOI: 10.3390/agriculture8100150

[48] Melesse A, Getye Y, Berihun K, Banerjee S. Effect of feeding graded levels of *Moringa stenopetala* leaf meal on growth performance, carcass traits and some serum biochemical parameters of Koekoek chickens. Livestock Science. 2013;**157**(2):498-505

[49] Habtemariam S. Investigation into the antioxidant and antidiabetic potential of *Moringa stenopetala:* Identification of the active principles. Natural Product Communications. 2015;**10**(3):475-478

[50] Makonnen E, Hunde A, Damecha G. Hypoglycaemic effect of *Moringa stenopetala* aqueous extract in rabbits. Phytotherapy Research. 1997;**11**(2):147-148

[51] Haji H, Mekonnen E, Debella A, Geleta B. Evaluation of diuretic and antihypertensive activity of leaf extracts of *Thymus schimperi* in rats. British Journal of Pharmacology and Toxicology. 2016;**7**(1):1-8. DOI: 10.19026/bjpt.7.2779

[52] Dadi DW, Emire SA, Hagos AD, Teka F, Woldekidan S, Abebe A, et al. Antihyperglycemic, vasodilator, and diuretic activities of microencapsulated bioactive product from *Moringa stenopetala* leaves extract. Journal of Food Quality. 2020;**2020**:1-8. DOI: 10.1155/2020/8882042

[53] Verma AR, Vijayakumar M, Mathela CS, Rao CV. In vitro and in vivo antioxidant properties of different fractions of *Moringa oleifera* leaves. Food and Chemical Toxicology. 2009;**47**(9):2196-2201

[54] Dadi DW, Emire SA, Hagos AD, Eun JB. Effect of ultrasound-assisted extraction of *Moringa stenopetala* leaves on bioactive compounds and their antioxidant activity. Food Technology and Biotechnology. 2019;**57**(1):77-86

[55] Toma A, Mekonnen E, Mekonnen Y, Debella A, Adisakwattana S. Antidiabetic activities of aqueous ethanol and

n-butanol fraction of *Moringa stenopetala* leaves in streptozotocin-induced diabetic rats. BMC Complementary and Alternative Medicine. 2015;**15**(1):242. DOI: 10.1186/s12906-015-0779-0

[56] Nardos A, Makonnen E, Debella A. Effects of crude extracts and fractions of *Moringa stenopetala (Baker f)* Cufodontis leaves in normoglycemic and alloxan-induced diabetic mice. African Journal of Pharmacy and Pharmacology. 2011;**5**(20):2220-2225

[57] Ghebreselassie D, Mekonnen Y, Gebru G, Ergete W, Huruy K. The effects of *Moringa stenopetala* on blood parameters and histopathology of liver and kidney in mice. Ethiopian Journal of Health Development. 2011;**25**(1):51-57. DOI: 10.4314/ejhd.v25i1.69850

[58] Shah S, Anjum S, Littler W. Use of diuretics in cardiovascular disease:(2) hypertension. Postgraduate Medical Journal. 2004;**80**(943):271-276. DOI: 10.1136/pgmj.2003.010843

[59] Versari D, Daghini E, Virdis A, Ghiadoni L, Taddei S. Endothelium-dependent contractions and endothelial dysfunction in human hypertension. British Journal of Pharmacology. 2009;**157**(4):527-536. DOI: 10.1111/j.1476-5381.2009.00240.x

[60] Mekonnen Y, Dräger B. Glucosinolates in *Moringa stenopetala*. Planta Medica. 2003;**69**(04):380-382. DOI: 10.1055/s-2003-38881

[61] Haile M, Duguma HT, Chameno G, Kuyu CG. Effects of location and extraction solvent on physico chemical properties of *Moringa stenopetala* seed oil. Heliyon. 2019;**5**(11):e02781. DOI: 10.1016/j.heliyon.2019.e02781

[62] Xu Y, Chen G, Guo M. Potential anti-aging components from *Moringa oleifera* leaves explored by affinity ultrafiltration with multiple drug targets. Frontiers in Nutrition. 2022;**9**:854882. DOI: 10.3389/fnut.2022.854882

[63] Melesse A. Comparative assessment on chemical compositions and feeding values of leaves of *Moringa stenopetala* and *Moringa oleifera* using in vitro gas production method. Journal of Applied Science and Technology. 2011;**2**(2):31-41

[64] Gidamis AB, Panga JT, Sarwatt SV, Chove BE, Shayo NB. Nutrient and antinutrient contents in raw and cooked young leaves and immature pods of *Moringa oleifera*. Ecology of Food and Nutrition. 2003;**42**(6):399-411

[65] Dadi DW, Emire SA, Hagos AD, Eun JB. Physical and functional properties, digestibility, and storage stability of spray- and freeze-dried microencapsulated bioactive products from *Moringa stenopetala* leaves extract. Industrial Crops and Products. 2020;**2020**:156. DOI: 10.1016/j.indcrop.2020.112891

[66] Seleshe S, Kang SN. *In vitro* antimicrobial activity of different solvent extracts from *Moringa stenopetala* leaves. Preventive Nutrition and Food Science. 2019;**24**(1):70-74. DOI: 10.3746/pnf.2019.24.1.70

Chapter 3

Nutritional and Functional Value of African Leafy Vegetables: Advantages and Limitations

Ntsoaki Joyce Malebo

Abstract

Globally, communities experience food insecurity, highlighting a need for access to food sources that are readily available with nutritional benefits. African leafy vegetables represent a plant-based food source that is rich in nutritional content and health benefits. These vegetables can grow unattended in the wild with minimal agricultural inputs which may negatively affect the environment, highlighting the advantages of their use. However, there is still a need to investigate the nutritional and functional value of these vegetables, focusing on their advantages and limitations before they can be recommended as an alternative food source. The chapter will focus on evaluating peer-reviewed journal articles, book chapters, and other publications to conduct a qualitative review.

Keywords: nutritional value, functional value, African leafy vegetables, plant-based diet, nutritional benefits

1. Introduction

The literature demonstrates that the Southern African Development Community (SADC) region is warming up faster than other regions in the global North prompting action towards adaptation strategies. The SADC region has observed adverse changes in rain patterns resulting in floods or multiple droughts. Reports by the Food Agriculture Organization [1] indicate the doubling of areas on the planet affected by droughts over a 40-year period [2]. The observed threat is a concern as the most vulnerable communities affected by high levels of unemployment, poverty, malnutrition, and inequality can be found in the SADC region. Studies indicate that climate change threatens health, ecology, and food security in sub-Saharan Africa [3, 4]. For ecology, an increase in woody vegetation has been observed which continues to replace indigenous habitats in certain regions [3]. The rise in temperatures leads to increased levels of evapotranspiration [5] which may affect food production and highlights the need to increase the propagation of climate-resilient crops such as African leafy vegetables (ALVs). Furthermore, because ALVs are considered climate-resilient crops, they can support climate adaptation strategies that are needed to address food insecurity [2]. Researchers [4] further argue that science interventions should be linked with local indigenous knowledge for adaptation and food security to address challenges such as climate change.

Maseko et al. [6] contend that the addition of ALVs in cropping systems can contribute to climate change adaptation strategies. This argument is supported by Nyathi et al. [7] who advocate for the diversification of current food production systems because vegetables such as Swiss chard which are available in commercial markets require high cultivation input whereas ALVs grow easily in the wild with minimal input from fertilizers and water. It has also been demonstrated that as climate changes, the presence of additional carbon dioxide in the air enhances the drought adaptation mechanisms of ALVs such as stomatal conductance which enables their growth during times of drought. This ensures the availability of highly nutritious vegetables which can support a plant-based diet.

Although commercially available C_3 vegetables such as Swiss chard increase biomass when carbon dioxide levels increase, their propagation requires high water input and fertilizers when compared to ALVs [8]. This indicates that such commercially available vegetables would not support climate adaptation strategies. Furthermore, an increase in carbon dioxide reportedly has a direct effect on nutrition as it reduces iron, zinc, and protein content in grains [4, 8], this implies that an increase in biomass may not result in high nutritional content. ALVs are recognized as a rich source of minerals and vitamins which are currently not available in commercially accessible vegetables [9–11]. Despite the known nutritional benefits of ALVs, urbanization, access to disposable income, and availability of commercial vegetables continue to influence changes in diet patterns in favor of commercial vegetables over ALVs [2]. In most African communities, ALVs are still regarded as weeds or food for the poor. Researchers argue that ALVs can be used in what is referred to as "hidden hunger" which is defined as micronutrient deficiencies [10, 12] observed globally due to a preference for ready-to-eat foods with limited nutritional value.

2. Methodology

A review of existing databases (Google Scholar, Science Direct, Web of Science, Scopus) was conducted for data published on ALVs from 2010 to 2023. Keywords such as "African leafy vegetables", "indigenous leafy vegetables", "nutritional value", and "functional value" were used to search for open access journal papers and book chapters. Inclusion criteria: Reviews and experimental papers published in peer-reviewed journals, book chapters, and conference proceedings between 2010 and 2023 were selected. Exclusion criteria: papers published prior to 2010 and not in peer-reviewed publications from sub-Saharan Africa. A total of 80 articles were retrieved and relevant papers were selected and used for the current review. Study limitations: The current study was limited to publications in peer-reviewed journals and book chapters, other studies published in non-peer-reviewed papers and also in other languages may have been excluded. The study also focused on ALVs mainly consumed in countries within sub-Sahara Africa and may have excluded leafy vegetables consumed in other parts of the African continent including the studied areas.

3. Type of African leafy vegetables (ALVs) consumed by communities

Different types of African leafy vegetables (ALVs) are consumed in various countries in sub-Saharan Africa. In Zimbabwe, ALVs such as *Cleome gynandra*, *Amaranthus thunbergii* Moq, *Vigna unguiculata*, *Corchorus tridens*, *Corchorus olitorius*, *Bidens pilosa*, and *Amaranthus hybridus* are consumed [13]. *Cleome gynandra* also known as African cabbage belongs to the family Capparaceae, an erect herb with palmately compound leaves (**Figure 1A**). *Amaranthus* species (**Figure 1B**), from the Amaranthaceae family, leaves are described as succulent and simple in some taxa. *Vigna unguiculata* is classified in the Leguminosae family and distinguished from other ALVs by tri-foliate leaves. *Corchorus* (**Figure 1C**) species belongs to the Tiliaceae family, with oblong to lanceolate leaves that have serrated margins and distinct hair-like teeth at the base. *B. pilosa* belongs to the family Asteraceae, differentiated by lobed, serrate, and opposite green leaves, and yellow or white flowers (**Figure 1D**).

According to [13], *C. gynandra* (Cleomaceae family) and *Vigna unguiculata* (Fabaceae family) are considered amongst the top five most important traditional vegetables in Zimbabwe. Although these vegetables are important traditional food sources, other species such as *B. pilosa* (Asteraceae family) are used not only as a food product but as medicine [14] based on the indigenous use of the plants. *B. pilosa* L. [15] is reportedly used to treat malaria, dysentery, diarrhea, and infected wounds or burns [16]. Most of these ALVs grow in the wild with minimal production input but [13] that vegetable species such as *C. gynadra* have been reportedly domesticated in home gardens and are purposely protected during activities such as digging, weeding, and land clearing due to the known benefits they provide.

Although ALVs grow in the wild, a study by [17] indicated that species such as *Amaranthus hybridus* and *C. gynandra* occur in all soil types, however, *C. gynandra*

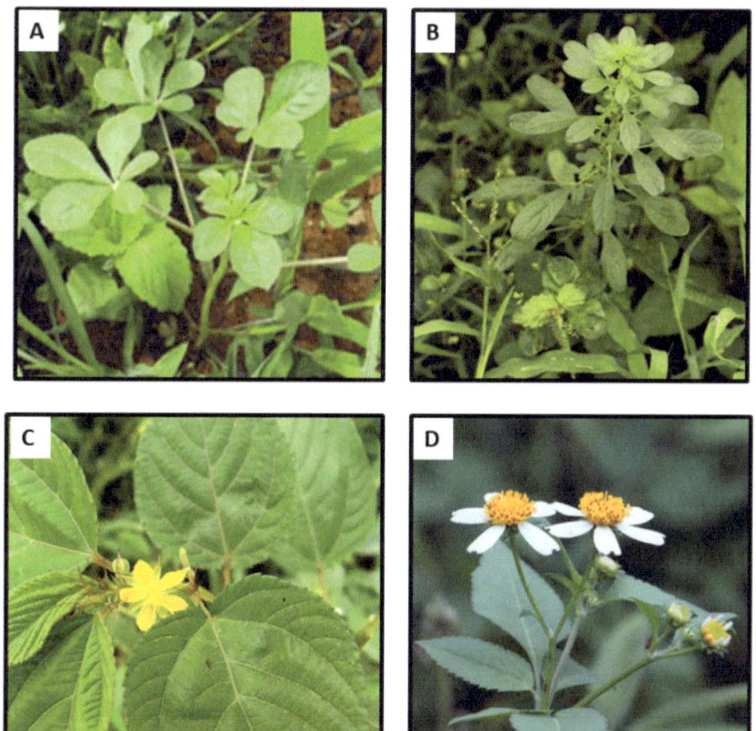

Figure 1.
An image showing selected ALVs. A – Cleome gynandra; B – Amaranthus thunbergii; C – Corchorus olitorius and D – Bidens pilosa.

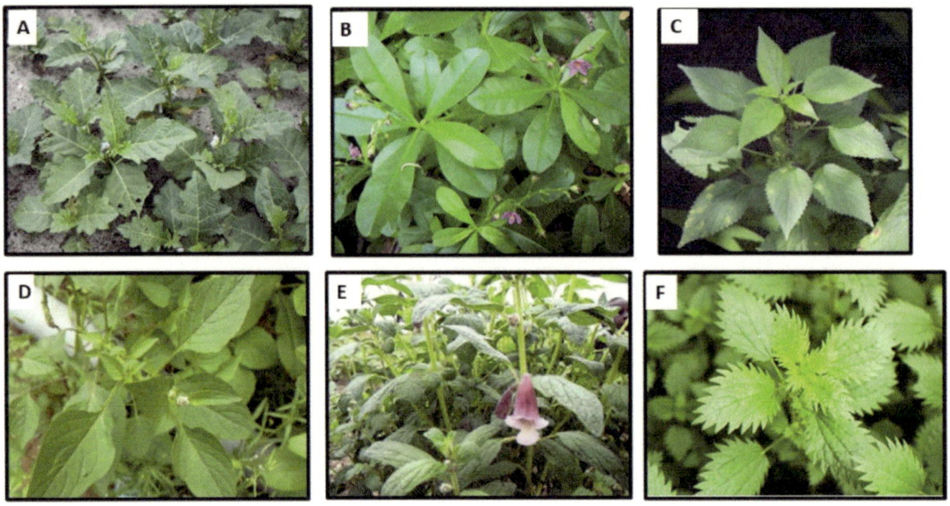

Figure 2.
An image of ALVs showing A – Solanum spp.; B – Talinum; C – Acalypha; D – Celosia; E – Sesammum; F – Urtica.

tends to be associated with sandy soils. Although *B. pilosa* reportedly thrives in any environment [14], it can be negatively affected by frost. Nightshade (*S. retroflexum* Dun.; Solanaceae family) leaves and tender shoots are consumed in most African countries [18]. African leafy vegetables mainly consumed in South Africa include *Amaranthus* species [6] such as *Amaranthus thunbergii* Moq., *Amaranthus spinosus* (L.) followed by *Corchorus* (*C. asplenifolius*, *Corchorus trilocularis*, *C. tridens* and *C. olitorius*), *Cleome monophylla* L. (*C. monophyla*, C. hirta) [19], *Vigna unguiculata,* and *Bidens pilosa* [20]. *Cleome gynandra*, *Curcubita maxima*, *Vigna unguiculata*, *Vigna unguiculata subsp. dekindtiana* var. *dekindtiana*, *V. unguiculate* subsp. *dekindtiana,* var. *huillensis*, *V. unguiculata* subsp. *rotracta*, *V. unguiculata* subsp. *stenophylla*, *V. unguiculate* subsp. *tenuis* var. *ovata*, *V. unguiculata* subsp. *unguiculata*, *Vigna unguiculata* subsp. *unguiculata, Solanum nigram*, *Urtica urens*, *Ribes uva crispa*, *Taraxacum officianale,* and *Beta vulgaris* [21] which are rich in nutrients, are also consumed in South Africa.

Solanum macrocarpon, *Talinum fruticosum*, *Corchorus* (**Figure 2**), and *Amaranthus* are consumed in Ghana [22]. In Côte d'Ivoire, although there are various ALVs consumed, the main reported vegetables include *Acalypha ciliate*, *Celosia trygina*, *Cleome gynandra*, *Solanum nigrum,* and *Sesammum radiatum*. In Southern Angola, *Bidens pilosa* and *Amaranth* are reported as the main ALVs consumed amongst the various vegetables reported [23]. The literature demonstrates that certain species from genera *Amaranth*, *Cleome*, *Bidens*, *Vigna*, *Solanum,* and *Corchorus* are readily available in most African communities. In most of these communities, although consumption continues to decrease, the nutritional benefits of the ALVs are recognized.

4. Nutritional benefits

African leafy vegetables are generally characterized by an abundance of carbohydrates, low protein, and fat content (**Table 1**). When consumed with high-calorie vegetables such as maize, supplementation for protein is needed to fully address malnutrition. Other studies have shown that adding peanut butter during cooking of ALVs enhances the presence of proteins and oils [26]. Generally, ALVs contain high amounts of flavonoids (**Table 1**) which are associated with health benefits such as protection against cardiovascular diseases, stroke, and cancer [22]. Additionally, ALVs contain moisture levels which are similar to commercially available leafy vegetables that are generally accepted by consumers [26]. The ash contents of *C. gynandra* and *Amaranth* [24] indicate that both vegetables may be good sources of minerals. The ALVs are considered sources of crude fiber which assists in the absorption of excess cholesterol.

Doue et al. [26] reported the presence of carotenoids in *Acalypha ciliate*, *Celosia trygina*, *Cleome gynandra*, *Solanum nigrum,* and *Sesammum radiatum* (**Table 1**). Although cooking methods may affect carotenoid content, the carotenoid content identified in these ALVs remains higher than what is reported for commercially available vegetables. Carotenoid pigments which include beta-carotene have high antioxidant properties which play an important role in reducing the occurrence of cancer. Additionally, vegetables with antioxidant properties can be used for the prevention of degenerative diseases [22]. African nightshade is one of the ALVs which reportedly

ALVs	Nutritional properties	References
Amaranthus spp.	Amino acids, Calcium, Carbohydrates, Carotenoids (β- carotene), Fiber, Flavonoids, Minerals (Copper, Iron, Magnesium, Potassium, Sodium, Sulfur and Zinc) and Phenolic compounds.	[7, 18, 22, 24, 25]
Acalypha ciliate	Flavonoids, Protein; Phenolic compounds,	[14, 22, 26]
Bidens pilosa	Carbohydrates, Calcium, Copper, Fiber, Flavonoids, Iron, Lipids, Minerals (Calcium, Copper, Iron, Magnesium, Manganese, Phosphorus, Sodium, Sulfur and Zinc), Phenolic compounds, Protein and Vitamins (A, E, C, beta-carotene)	[14, 18, 23]
Celosia trygina	Amino acids; Ascorbic acid, Carotenoids, Flavonoids and Phenolic compounds.	[23, 26]
Cleome gynandra	Carotenoids, Calcium, Flavonoids, Glucosinolates, Iron, Magnesium, Manganese, Protein, Phenolic compounds, Potassium, Phosphorus, and Zinc	[7, 14, 22, 25–27]
Corchorus olitorius	Calcium, Carbohydrates, Copper, Fiber, Flavonoids, Iron, Magnesium, Phenols, Protein and Zinc	[20, 22]
Sesammum radiatum	Amino acids, Carbohydrates, Carotenoids, Fiber, Flavonoids, Minerals, Phenolic compounds	[14, 22, 24, 26]
Solanum spp.	Carbohydrate, Calcium, Carotenoids, Copper, Fat, Fiber, Flavonoids, Iron, Minerals (potassium manganese), Protein, Vitamins (Folate, Vitamin A, Riboflavin and Thiamine) Phenolic compounds	[10, 12, 14, 18, 20, 22, 26, 28]
Talinum fruticosum	Carbohydrates, β-carotene, Fiber, Flavonoids, Minerals (calcium, magnesium potassium), Phenolic compounds, Proteins Vitamin C and E	[22]
Vigna unguiculata	Carbohydrates, Carotenoids, Flavonoids, Phenolic compounds, Protein	[13, 25]

Table 1.
Nutritional composition of selected ALVs.

serves as a rich source of minerals such as potassium, manganese, and vitamins in the form of Vitamin A and folate [18]. Other studies indicate that African nightshade is a source of protein, minerals, and beta-carotene which is reportedly higher than commonly consumed vegetables [10, 12, 29]. Other vitamins identified in African nightshade include thiamine, riboflavin, and folate [12, 28].

Amaranth is recognized as a good source of pro-vitamin A [25] which are carotenoids that the body convert to vitamin A. Potassium, calcium, magnesium, phosphorus, iron, manganese, and zinc were identified in high amounts in *Cleome* leaf tissue [27]. Vitamins such as beta-carotene, vitamin A, vitamin C and medium in vitamin E and protein have also been reported in blackjack [14]. Minerals identified in blackjack include calcium, phosphorus, sodium, manganese, copper, zinc, magnesium, and iron [14]. The minerals are beneficial for human health with iron playing an important role in blood production [18]. The presence of high carbohydrate content in leafy vegetables indicates a high caloric content, a study conducted by [22] showed a high carbohydrate content in dried *Solanum macrocarpon, Talinum fruticosum*, *Corchorus olitorius* and *Amaranthus* spp. when compared to other studies. Crude fiber was observed by [22] in dried *Solanum macrocarpon*, *Talinum fruticosum*, *Corchorus olitorius,* and *Amaranthus*; the study further showed that these dried ALVs are good sources of protein. However, other studies observed minimal amounts [26] of protein in ALVs.

5. Functional properties

Various studies have demonstrated that traditional leafy vegetables possess phenols (gallic acid) and flavonoids which grant these vegetables various functional properties. Obeng [22] showed that *Solanum macrocarpon*, *Talinum fruticosum*, *Corchorus olitorius,* and *Amaranthus* spp. possess phenols and flavonoids. Obeng [22] reported antioxidant properties when dried *Solanum macrocarpon*, *Talinum fruticosum*, *Corchorus olitorius,* and *Amaranthus* spp. were assessed. Although antioxidant properties were identified, the study reported that high quantities of ALVs and frequent consumption are recommended to provide consumers with the reported health benefits. Nightshade possesses antioxidant properties due to the presence of phenolic metabolites [18, 30]. Jiménez-Aguilar and Grusak [31] demonstrated that some *Amaranth* species possess antioxidant properties which are higher than properties reported in spider flower (**Table 2**), African nightshade, and spinach. Although additional studies are needed, [14] have reported that blackjack possesses antioxidant properties. The health benefits of vegetables with antioxidant properties have been demonstrated.

Blackjack possesses various chemical compounds such as astragalin, a flavonoid found in various plants, reportedly has anticandidal activity. The compound was shown to inhibit fungous biofilm development. Kissanga et al. [23] indicate that *A. hybridus* is used for medicinal properties in Angola. Antibacterial properties of blackjack against gram-negative *E. coli* as well as antifungal properties have been reported [14]. In addition to the identified antimicrobial properties, blackjack has been used to treat various diseases such as indigestion, diarrhea, dysentery, wounds, and respiratory infections [14]. One of the bioactive compounds, astragalin, isolated from blackjack reportedly has anti-parasite properties against *Trigonoscuta cruzi* [14]; it affects the growth of the parasite by changing the morphology of the cell membrane.

Mtenga and Ripanda [14] also report that blackjack possesses anti-inflammatory properties due to the presence of squalene. Mokganya and Tshisikhawe [15] further

African leafy vegetables	Functional properties	Compounds	References
Amaranthus	Antioxidant and anti-inflammatory	Quercetin-3-glycosides	[20, 25]
	Antioxidant, antitumor, anti-inflammatory, antimicrobial, and antidiabetic activity	Hydroxycinnamic acid derivatives	[25]
	Antioxidant, anti-inflammatory, and antimicrobial	Kaempferol-3-rutinoside (nicotiflorin)	[18, 25]
Bidens spp	Anticandidal Antibacterial and antifungal Antimicrobial Antibacterial, antioxidant, and Antifungal Anti-inflammatory B-caryophyllene and s-cadinene	Astragalin Axillaroside Iso-Vanillin Daucene Squalene Antioxidant	[14]
Cleome spp	Antioxidant and anti-inflammatory	Quercetin glycosides	[20, 27]
	Antioxidant and anti-inflammatory	Kaempferol and isorhamnetin diglycosides	[25, 27]
Corchorus spp	Antioxidant	Quercetin glycosides	[20]
	Antimicrobial and antioxidant	Glucoronic acid	
	Antimicrobial	Galacturonic acid	
Solanum spp	Antioxidant, antitumor, anti-inflammatory, antimicrobial, and antidiabetic activity	Hydroxycinnamic acid derivatives	[25]
	Antioxidant, anti-inflammatory, anti-obesity, and anti-diabetic	Chlorogenic acids	[12, 18]
	Antioxidant, anti-inflammatory, and antimicrobial	Kaempferol derivatives, rhamnetin, and rutin	[18]
	Antioxidant, anti-inflammatory, anti-allergy, and anti-tumor activity	Quercetin glycosides	[18]
V. unguiculata	Antimicrobial, antiviral, anti-inflammatory, antidiabetic, antioxidant	Coumaroyl derivatives	[25]
	Antioxidant, anti-inflammatory, and antimicrobial	Quercetin and kaempferol	[18, 28]

Table 2.
Functional properties of selected African leafy vegetables.

indicate that liquid extracted from blackjack has been used to treat inflammation and wounds as it contains antimicrobial compounds such as Iso-Vanillin and Daucene. Similar properties were reported in nightshade due to the presence of phenolic metabolites such as chlorogenic acids [18, 32]. *C. gynandra,* which is commonly used by various African communities, is characterized by compounds such as quercetin glycosides that possess anti-inflammatory properties, and claims by communities indicate that decoctions are consumed orally to reduce blood pressure [15]. Other commonly used ALVs such as *S. retroflexum* L. are reportedly used to treat earache in young children [15] because the ALV contains hydroxycinnamic acid derivatives with antimicrobial and anti-inflammatory properties (**Table 2**). *V. unguiculata* L. is used to treat stomach problems [15] because it possesses compounds (Coumaroyl derivatives) with anti-inflammatory and anti-microbial properties. Researchers reported antidiabetic, anti-obesity, and antihypertensive properties of *B. pilosa* worldwide, indicating the possibility of its application in the mitigation of diabetes, hypertension, and obesity.

6. Advantages

It is generally accepted that ALV is resistant to drought, pests, and diseases when compared to commercially available vegetables [6, 10]. Some communities are consuming ALVs as an important resource for climate adaptation strategies [12, 33] and for food security. Kissanga and others [23] reported that vegetables are used by communities during droughts because ALVs are resistant to environmental changes. The morphology of some of the ALVs such as leaves with a waxy cuticle observed in *Amaranthus* spp. protects the vegetable against rapid moisture loss. African leafy vegetables such as *Amaranthus*, *Brassica nigra*, and *Cleome gynandra* are also drought hardy because of their excellent stomatal conductance. Some ALV species such as *Bidens pilosa* have an extraordinary recovery rate after experiencing prolonged drought periods [20].

ALVs grow in the wild with low input from pesticides and fertilizers. Additionally, bioactive compounds such as alkaloids from *Bidens pilosa* can be used as organic pesticides which are environmentally friendly and biodegradable [14]; compounds from blackjack can be used to control fungal pathogens and weeds which affect plant growth. Doue et al. [26] have reported that ALVs can serve as fertilizers as they improve the growth of other plants by improving soil fertility. Economic opportunities exist to include ALVs such as *Amaranth* in bread products, the advantages of this type of postharvest processing not only provides communities with a source of nutritious bread but increases the need and value of these vegetables [2] and also provides an opportunity to sell a highly nutritious product.

7. Limitations

Despite the added advantages of ALVs, there are some limitations that affect their use. African leafy vegetables are highly perishable, and preparation and preservation approaches affect their long-term nutritional quality [6]. Preparation methods at high temperatures can affect compounds such as vitamins and minerals. This can have a negative effect on some of the reported health benefits of ALVs. Other studies indicate that alternative methods for preparation are needed and supplementation with other sources of protein and fat may be necessary to enhance the nutritional benefits of ALVs with low fat and protein content. Doue et al. [26] argue that preparation of ALV with red palm oil may enhance the availability of vitamin A which is needed to address deficiencies that are reported in the sub-Saharan region. Although steaming reduces the nutritional properties in other ALVs, [18] demonstrated that this process can significantly reduce anti-nutritive compounds in nightshade, making it the most suitable processing method. Similar studies have shown that post-harvest processes can also be beneficial and assist with the release of complex minerals, enhancing bioavailability and bioactivity [12, 34].

Lack of post-harvest processing of vegetables was reported to result in loss of quantitative, nutritive, and economic value of nightshade along the supply chain [35]. Similar losses were observed in other ALVs such as *Cleome gynandra* L., *African nightshade,* and *Amaranthus* spp. Gogo and others [35] demonstrated in their study that loss due to pests and diseases occurred mainly postharvest and this is influenced by various factors which include transport of vegetables in suitable conditions, packaging, and poor handling. African leafy vegetables are highly perishable [10] and to date, different methods to prolong their shelf life are explored. Lactic acid fermentation [36] is a method commonly used by African communities which prevents the growth of spoilage microbes and increases the sensory and shelf life properties of vegetables. Although postharvest value addition opportunities exist for ALVs, their availability in small quantities affects the possibility of establishing their availability in the food production chain [2].

Poor seed quality limits propagation and affects yield which results in a focus on exotic plants rather than African leafy vegetables [20]. Stoll and others [10] have also reported poor seed quality as one of the factors which influences the availability and consumption of ALVs. The challenge continues to exist due to limited investment in research and development [12, 21, 37]. These challenges are intensified by the presence of heavy metals in ALVs due to contamination of soils. This is a concern that studies indicate may affect the advocacy and use of these vegetables [23]. The presence of antinutritional compounds such as cyanogenic glycosides, oxalates, phytates, nitrates, and tannins is one of the challenges identified that discourages the use of ALVs. However, the implementation of suitable agro-processing techniques to facilitate the elimination of antinutritive compounds should be further explored [12] if the use of ALVs is going to be promoted. Addressing the presence of antinutritional properties of ALVs is important because their presence influences the absorption of vitamins and minerals present in vegetables, reducing their value. The biggest challenge which affects the use of ALVs is the unsustainable harvesting because the vegetables are not formally cultivated [6].

Consumer acceptability and perceptions about ALVs have generally influenced their limited consumption and propagation. The availability of mainstream vegetables influences the consumption and propagation of ALVs [38]. Blackjack (*Biden pilosa*) is underutilized in sub-Saharan Africa due to its classification as a weed or a wild plant, which creates a negative perception in the community concerning the consumption of wild or weed plants [14]. The use of blackjack despite its identified benefits is hindered by its categorization as inversive species (weeds). The perceptions that exist in communities affect the marketing of ALVs as an alternative source of nutrition. There is a general agreement that ALVs are poorly marketed [10] despite the nutritional and medicinal properties known by indigenous people. According to [21], information about the economic value of ALV is lacking. ALVs are perceived as foods with low social status and only meant for the poor by certain communities [25, 39]. Young consumers still prefer Western-based diets which are widely promoted on media platforms and represent a higher-class status within their communities. But [36] have reported that in Kenya, consumer awareness about the nutritional benefits of ALVs has resulted in an increase in their use.

8. Conclusions

The current review has demonstrated the advantages of using ALVs as part of a plant-based diet, however, awareness about the nutritional and medicinal benefits of ALVs is still needed to change current consumer perceptions and preferences. Most of the ALVs discussed have micronutrients which can be used to address the challenge of hunger. Their sale by communities can contribute to socio-economic development [18] and address the goal of ending poverty in the sub-Saharan region and hidden hunger globally. Research is still needed to assess the bioavailability of nutritional compounds and their benefits following digestion to recommend their use in plant-based diets. The ability of the vegetables to withstand adverse climatic conditions and growth with minimal water and pesticide input was also demonstrated. This highlights the continuous availability of ALVs despite climate change challenges. The way forward would be the development of policies that advocate for and promote the use of ALVs as proposed elsewhere [12]. Although fermentation has been used as an effective method to prolong the shelf life of ALVs, sensory evaluation studies indicate consumer acceptance of fermented vegetables is minimal. This highlights the need to continuously investigate various postharvest preservation methods to protect this valuable nutritional resource for plant-based diets.

Acknowledgements

The author would like to thank the Central University of Technology, Free State, the South African National Research Foundation (NRF), and the Southern African Science Service Centre for Climate Change and Adaptive Land Management (SASSCAL) for supporting the work conducted in this study.

Conflict of interest

"The authors declare no conflict of interest."

Author details

Ntsoaki Joyce Malebo
Central University of Technology, Free State, Bloemfontein, South Africa

*Address all correspondence to: nmalebo@cut.ac.za

References

[1] FAO. Food and Agriculture Organization of the United Nations Infographic: Drought & Agriculture. Rome, Italy: FAO; 2017

[2] Noort MWJ, Renzetti S, Linderhof V, du Rand GE, Marx-Pienaar NJMM, de Kock HL, et al. Towards sustainable shifts to healthy diets and food security in sub-Saharan Africa with climate-resilient crops in bread-type products: A food system analysis. Food. 2022;**11**:135. DOI: 10.3390/foods11020135

[3] Vukeya L, Mokotjomela TM, Malebo NJ, Smith DAE, Oke S. The vegetation cover dynamics and potential drivers of habitat change over 30 years in the Free State National Botanical Garden, South Africa. Regional Environmental Change. 2023;**23**:24. DOI: 10.1007/s10113-022-02024-9

[4] Amoak D, Luginaah I, McBean G. Climate change, food security, and health: Harnessing agroecology to build climate-resilient communities. Sustainability. 2022;**14**:13954. DOI: 10.3390/su142113954

[5] Ruzvidzo S. Effects of Evapotranspiration on Water Quantity and Quality along the Modder River Catchment Using Remote Sensing. South Africa: Central University of Technology, Free State; 2021

[6] Maseko I, Mabhaudhi T, Tesfay S, Araya HT, Fezzehazion M, Du Plooy CP. African leafy vegetables: A review of status, production and utilization in South Africa. Sustainability. 2018;**10**:16. DOI: 10.3390/su10010016

[7] Nyathi MK, van Halsema GE, Annandale JG, Struik PC. Calibration and validation of the AquaCrop model for repeatedly harvested leafy vegetables grown under different irrigation regimes. Agricultural Water Management. 2018;**208**:107-119. DOI: 10.1016/j.agwat.2018.06.012

[8] Lloyd SJ, Kovats RS, Chalabi Z. Climate change, crop yields, and undernutrition: Development of a model to quantify the impact of climate scenarios on child undernutrition. Environmental Health Perspective. 2011;**119**:1817. DOI: 10.1289/ehp.1003311

[9] Mungofa N, Sibanyoni JJ, Mashau ME, Beswa D. Prospective role of indigenous leafy vegetables as functional food ingredients. Molecules. 2022;**27**:7995. DOI: 10.3390/molecules27227995

[10] Stoll DA, Wafula EN, Mathara JM, Trierweiler B, Kulling SE, Huch M. Fermentation of African nightshade leaves with lactic acid bacterial starter cultures. International Journal of Food Microbiology. 2021;**342**:109056. DOI: 10.1016/j.ijfoodmicro.2021.109056

[11] Wafula EN, Franz CMAP, Rohn S, Huch M, Mathara JM, Trierweiler B. Fermentation of African indigenous leafy vegetables to lower postharvest losses, maintain quality and increase product safety. African Journal of Horticultural Science. 2016;**9**:1-13

[12] Sultanbawa Y, Sivakumar D. Enhanced nutritional and phytochemical profiles of selected underutilized fruits, vegetables, and legumes. Current Opinion in Food Science. 2022;**46**:100853. DOI: 10.1016/j.cofs.2022.100853

[13] Maroyi A. Use of weeds as traditional vegetables in Shurugwi District, Zimbabwe. Journal of Ethnobiology

and Ethnomedicine. 2013;**9**:60. DOI: 10.1186/1746-4269-9-60

[14] Mtenga DV, Ripanda SA. A review on the potential of underutilized Blackjack (*Biden pilosa*) naturally occurring in sub-Saharan Africa. Heliyon. 2022;**8**:e09586. DOI: 10.1016/j.heliyon.2022.e09586

[15] Mokganya MG, Tshisikhawe MP. Medicinal uses of selected wild edible vegetables consumed by Vhavenda of the Vhembe District Municipality, South Africa. South African Journal of Botany. 2019;**122**:184-188. DOI: 10.1016/j.sajb.2018.09.029

[16] Arthur GD, Naidoo KK, Coopoosamy RM. *Bidens pilosa* L.: Agricultural and pharmaceutical importance. Journal of Medicinal Plants Research. 2012;**6**:3282-3287. DOI: 10.5897/jmpr12.195

[17] Macheka L, Manditsera FA, Ngadzec RT, Mubaiwa J, Nyarugwe S, Bangirae C, et al. Agro-ecological distribution and consumption of wild harvested edible insects, fruits, and vegetables in rural Zimbabwe. Future Foods. 2022;**6**:100187. DOI: 10.1016/j.fufo.2022.100187

[18] Managa MG, Mpaia S, Remizeb F, Garciab C, Sivakumara D. Impact of moist cooking methods on colour, anti-nutritive compounds, and phenolic metabolites in African nightshade (*Solanum retroflexum* Dun.). Food Chemistry. 2020;**325**:126805. DOI: 10.1016/j.foodchem.2020.126805

[19] Rankoana SA. Indigenous plant foods of Dikgale community in South Africa. Journal of Ethnic Foods. 2021;**8**:5. DOI: 10.1186/s42779-021-00080-w

[20] Shayanowako AIT, Morrissey O, Tanzi A, Muchuweti M, Mendiondo GM, Mayes S, et al. African leafy vegetables for improved human nutrition and food system resilience in Southern Africa: A scoping review. Sustainability. 2021;**13**:2896. DOI: 10.3390/su13052896

[21] Mbhenyane XG. Indigenous foods and their contribution to nutrient requirements. South African Journal of Clinical Nutrition. 2017;**30**(4):5-7

[22] Obeng E, Kpodoa FM, Tettey CO, Essumana EK, Adzinyo OA. Antioxidant, total phenols, and proximate constituents of four tropical leafy vegetables. Scientific African. 2020;**7**:e00227. DOI: 10.1016/j.sciaf.2019.e00227

[23] Kissanga AR, Sales J, Moldão M, Alves V, Mendes H, Romeiras MM, et al. Nutritional and functional properties of wild leafy vegetables for improving food security in Southern Angola. Frontiers in Sustainable Food Systems. 2021;**5**:791705. DOI: 10.3389/fsufs.2021.791705

[24] Ntuli NR. Nutrient content of scarcely known wild leafy vegetables from northern KwaZulu-Natal, South Africa. South African Journal of Botany. 2019;**127**:19-24. DOI: 10.1016/j.sajb.2019.08.033

[25] Neugart S, Baldermann S, Ngwene B, Wesonga J, Schreiner M. Indigenous leafy vegetables of Eastern Africa — A source of extraordinary secondary plant metabolites. Food Research International. 2017;**100**:411-422. DOI: 10.1016/j.foodres.2017.02.014

[26] Doue G, Vanie BIG, Zoue LT, Megnanou RM, Zouzou M. Assessment of the nutritional value of spontaneous leafy vegetables of interest from Marahoue (Cote D'Ivoire) region and their traditional homemade sauces. Agronomie Africaine Sp. 2021;**33**(2):227-238

[27] Omondi EO, Engels C, Nambafu G, Schreiner M, Neugart S,

Abukutsa-Onyangod M, et al. Nutritional compound analysis and morphological characterization of spider plant (*Cleome gynandra*) - an African indigenous leafy vegetable. Food Research International. 2017;**100**:284-295. DOI: 10.1016/j.foodres.2017.06.050

[28] Sangija F, Martin H, Matemu A. African nightshades (*Solanum nigrum* complex): The potential contribution to human nutrition and livelihoods in sub-Saharan Africa. Comprehensive Reviews in Food Science and Food Safety. 2021;**20**:3284-3318. DOI: 10.1111/1541-4337.12756

[29] Ronald M, Kebede SW, Bokelmann W. Protein and energy contribution of African indigenous vegetables: Evidence from selected rural and peri-urban counties of Kenya. African Journal of Food, Agriculture, Nutrition and Development. 2020;**20**:15177-15193. DOI: 10.18697/ajfand.89.17515

[30] Yuan B, Byrnes D, Giurleo D, Villani T, Simon JE, Wu Q. Rapid screening of toxic glycoalkaloids and micronutrients in edible nightshades (*Solanum* spp.). Journal of Food and Drug Analysis. 2018;**26**:751-760. DOI: 10.1016/j.jfda.2017.10.005

[31] Jiménez-Aguilar DM, Grusak MA. Minerals, vitamin C, phenolics, flavonoids and antioxidant activity of *Amaranthus* leafy vegetables. Journal of Food Composition and Analysis. 2017;**58**:33-39. DOI: 10.1016/j.jfca.2017.01.005

[32] Park YS, Namiesnik J, Vearasilp K, Leontowicz H, Leontowicz M, Gorinstein S. Bioactive compounds, and the antioxidant capacity in new kiwi fruit cultivars. Food Chemistry. 2014;**165**:354-361. DOI: 10.1016/j.foodchem.2014.05.114

[33] Chimonyo VGP, Wimalasiri EM, Kunz R, Modi AT, Tafadzwanashe M. Optimizing traditional cropping systems under climate change: A case of maize landraces and bambara groundnut. Front Sustain Food System. 2020;**4**:1-19. DOI: 10.3389/fsufs.2020.562568

[34] Troesch B, Biesalski HK, Bos R, Buskens E, Calder PC, Saris WHM, et al. Increased intake of foods with high nutrient density can help to break the intergenerational cycle of malnutrition and obesity. Nutrients. 2015;7:6016-6037. DOI: 10.3390/nu7075266

[35] Gogo EO, Opiyob AM, Ulrichsa C, Huyskens-Keila S. Nutritional and economic postharvest loss analysis of African indigenous leafy vegetables along the supply chain in Kenya. Postharvest Biology and Technology. 2017;**130**:39-47. DOI: 10.1016/j.postharvbio.2017.04.007

[36] Misci C, Taskin E, et al. Fermentation as a tool for increasing food security and nutritional quality of indigenous African leafy vegetables: The case of *Cucurbita* sp. Food Microbiology. 2021;**99**:103820. DOI: 10.1016/j.fm.2021.103820

[37] Minnis P, editor. New Lives for Ancient and Extinct Crops. Tucson, AZ, USA: University of Arizona Press; 2014

[38] Salami SO, Adegbajub OD, Idrisc OA, Jimohd MO, Olatunjic TL, Omononae S, et al. South African wild fruits and vegetables under a changing climate: The implications on health and economy. South African Journal of Botany. 2022;**145**:13-27. DOI: 10.1016/j.sajb.2021.08.038

[39] Dwebaa TP, Mearns MA. Conserving indigenous knowledge as the key to the current and future use of traditional vegetables. International Journal of Information Management. 2011;**31**:564-571. DOI: 10.1016/j.ijinfomgt.2011.02.009

Section 2

Bioactive Compounds from Vegetal Sources

Chapter 4

Beneficial Effects of Extra Virgin Olive Oil Rich in Phenolic Compounds on Cardiovascular Health

Imen Ghorbel, Mariem Chaâbane, Naziha Grati Kammoun and Najiba Zeghal

Abstract

The Mediterranean diet (Med-diet) includes a high consumption of cereals, fruits, legumes and vegetables, a moderate fish intake and a low consumption of red meat. Olive oil is a basic component of the Med-diet due to its numerous health benefits. In the last decade, many epidemiological studies have confirmed the protective role of extra virgin olive oil (EVOO) against several chronic illnesses including cardiovascular diseases. EVOO is mainly composed of triacylglycerols, with oleic acid as the dominating esterified fatty acid, and other minor compounds. Among them, phenolic compounds, such as hydroxytyrosol and its derivatives (oleuropein and tyrosol), are the principal components responsible for the cardioprotective effects. They are endowed with wide biological activities, including strong antioxidant properties, allowing the prevention of cardiovascular risk factors, such as atherosclerosis, plasma lipid disorders, endothelial dysfunction, hypertension, obesity and type 2 diabetes. The aim of the present chapter was to elucidate the beneficial effect of EVOO, as part of the Mediterranean-style diets, on cardiovascular risk factors and to discuss the underlying mechanisms by which polyphenols exert their effects.

Keywords: olive oil, phenolic compounds, cardiovascular diseases, endothelial dysfunction, atherosclerosis, type 2 diabetes mellitus

1. Introduction

The Mediterranean diet (Med-diet) is beneficial for the human health as it provides for the consumer foods rich in biological active substances. It is composed of fish, unsaturated fats, whole grains, fruits and vegetables, nuts and legumes. Olive oil has been traditionally used as the main fat in the Mediterranean regions, and recently, it has become more popular worldwide. Extra virgin olive oil (EVOO) is obtained from the fruit of the olive tree by mechanical or other physical means as follows: washing, decantation or centrifugation, and filtration. A Med-diet rich in olive oil supplies an average of 10–20 mg of phenols per day [1]. The lipophilic fraction represents 90.0–99.0% of EVOO and it is mainly composed of phospholipids and triacylglycerols, while the hydrophilic fraction (0.5–1.5%) contains hydrocarbons, aliphatic alcohols, sterols, pigments, and several volatile and phenolic compounds [2]. Phenols are the organic molecules characterized by the existence of a hydroxyl group attached directly to the benzene ring. The major classes of phenolic compounds present in olive oil are phenolic acids, phenolic alcohols, secoiridoids, and flavonoids [3]. They have the capacity to donate the hydrogen atom of the phenolic hydroxyl group to free radicals. Hydroxytyrosol (HT), one of the main phenolic compounds of EVOO, reduces oxidative stress by improving lipid profile and inhibiting inflammatory cells [4]. The wide biological activities of HT are associated with its strong antioxidant and radical-scavenging activities [5]. HT and oleuropein, another major phenolic component of EVOO, are potent scavengers of hydroxyl radicals ($OH^{\cdot}$), peroxynitrite (ONOOH), and superoxide radicals ($O_2^{\cdot-}$) [5]. Phenols are able to modulate redox status through direct action on enzymes, proteins and different signaling pathways. The oxidative stress process plays a crucial role in the development of cardiovascular diseases (CVDs). It contributes to the pathogenesis of atherosclerosis, endothelial dysfunction, plasma lipid disorders and hypertension. It has been reported that EVOO has beneficial effects on cardiovascular risk factors, such as coagulation, platelet aggregation, fibrinolysis, endothelial dysfunction and lipid metabolism alteration [6]. Moreover, EVOO shows potential actions on markers of inflammation related to CVD, such as interleukin 6 and C-reactive protein [7].

The aim of the present chapter was to present some evidence from previous studies demonstrating the beneficial effect of EVOO, as part of the Mediterranean-style diets, on cardiovascular risk factors, namely atherosclerosis, plasma lipid disorders, endothelial dysfunction, hypertension, obesity and type 2 diabetes mellitus (T2D), and to discuss the underlying mechanisms by which polyphenols exert their effects.

2. Phenolic compounds present in EVOO

In olive oil, both simple and complex phenolic compounds contribute to its stability and affect its sensory properties. Polyphenols are a large and heterogeneous group of phytochemicals containing phenol rings. According to Bajoub et al. [3], the most abundant phenolic compounds can be classified according to their chemical structure as follows: secoiridoids (oleuropein, oleuropein aglycone, oleocanthol), simple phenols (tyrosol, HT), lignans (pinoresinol, syringaresinol), flavonoids (luteolin, apigenin) and phenolic acids (**Figure 1**). It has been demonstrated that the variability of those phenols can be related to a combination of agronomic and technological processes [8]. Indeed, once ingested, olive oil polyphenols give rise to different metabolites which are able to reach tissues and exert their beneficial effects [9]. Natural phenols have been demonstrated to modulate cell redox status through direct actions on enzymes, proteins, receptors and different signaling pathways [10, 11].

3. EVOO polyphenols and CVD

In recent years, several studies have demonstrated the cardiovascular health benefits associated with the regular consumption of olive oil with a high polyphenol content. Hence, understanding the mechanisms contributing to the favorable effect

DOI: http://dx.doi.org/10.5772/intechopen.104883

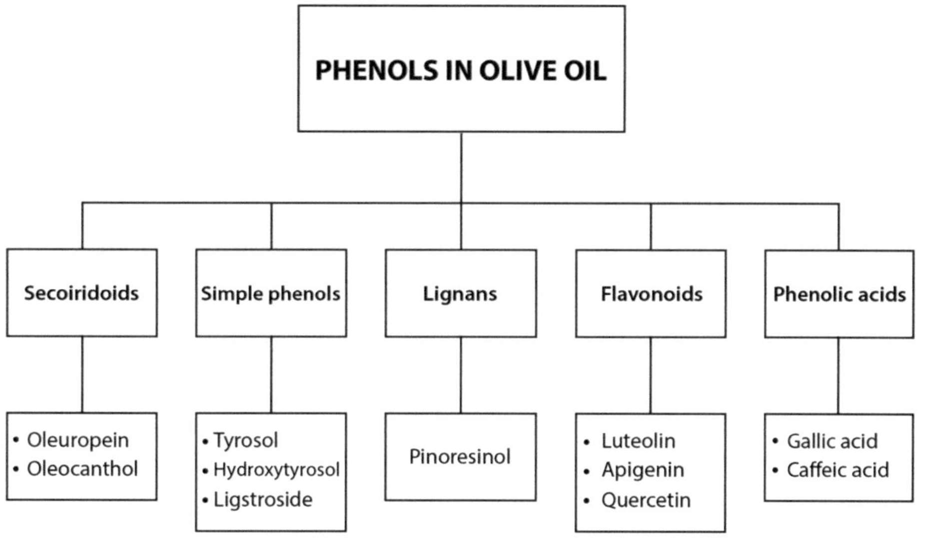

Figure 1.
The phenolic compounds present in olive oil.

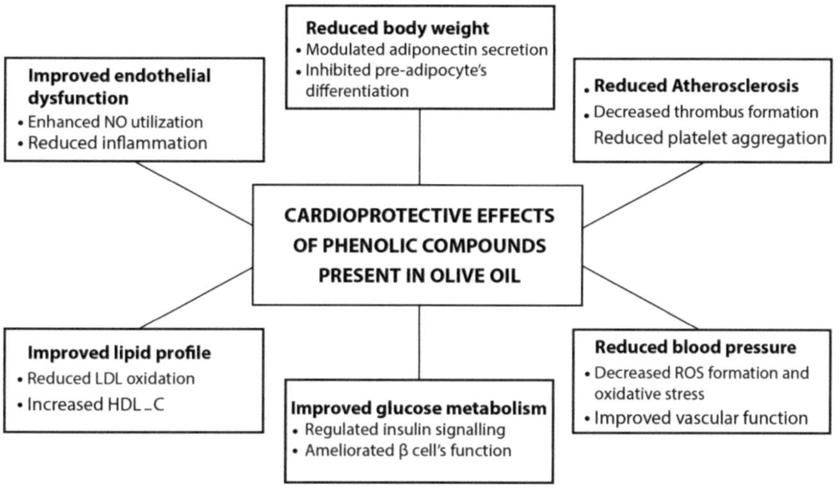

Figure 2.
Cardioprotective effects of phenolic compounds present in olive oil.

of these bioactive compounds is of crucial importance. In this setting, the main mechanisms responsible for the cardioprotective effects of olive oil polyphenols against atherosclerosis, plasma lipid disorders, endothelial dysfunction, hypertension, obesity and T2D will be reviewed (**Figure 2**).

3.1 Polyphenols and atherosclerosis

It has been known that several CVD are directly related to thrombus formation [12]. The oxidative stress process, an imbalance between reactive oxygen species

(ROS) production and endogenous antioxidant defense system, plays a crucial role in the development of heart diseases. An excessive production of ROS causes oxidative damage to the vascular endothelium [13] by promoting vascular cells proliferation, apoptosis, and necrosis which may result in the formation of atherosclerotic plaques leading to thrombosis [13, 14]. The uncontrolled ROS formation alters the vascular tone, which is mediated by a decrease of nitric oxide (NO) bioavailability, the most potent endogenous vasodilator [15]. A low NO level is associated with the promotion of platelet aggregation, adhesion of inflammatory cells and fibrinolysis which are responsible for the developmental process of atherosclerotic plaques [16]. Olive oil intake contributes to the homeostasis of the thrombogenic profile by improving the production of coagulation factors and biomarkers related to platelet aggregation [17]. Oleuropein and HT have been shown to exert several protective effects *in vivo* on a model of atherosclerosis inhibiting endothelial activation and monocyte-endothelial cell adhesion [18]. Besides, these simple phenolic compounds have been described as the potent inhibitors of platelet aggregation in several *in vitro* experiments [19].

3.2 Polyphenols and plasma lipid disorders

Plasma total cholesterol (TC), low density lipoprotein cholesterol (LDL-C) and high-density lipoprotein cholesterol (HDL-C) levels are included in CVD risk assessment tools. The elevated levels of TC and LDL-C have been considered as risk factors for atherosclerosis, which is the primary cause of CVD. LDL-C is the main carrier of circulating cholesterol to the target vascular cells. Consequently, circulating LDL-C is a valuable indicator of the amount of lipid accumulation in the arterial wall. Their oxidation is considered to be the triggering factor for the biochemical processes leading to atherosclerotic plaque formation in the sub-endothelial space [20]. Apolipoprotein B (Apo B) is the primary protein component of LDL-C, while apolipoprotein A (Apo A) is the primary protein component of HDL-C. Polyphenols affect apolipoproteins (Apo) A and B, modify LDL-C particles, and reduce plasma triglyceride (TG) levels by increasing the lipoprotein lipase activity, which decreases LDL-C concentrations in the blood circulation [21, 22]. The mechanism by which polyphenols reduce hepatic Apo B production relies on their binding with the plasma membrane transport P-glycoprotein, which inhibits cholesterol esterification [23]. The administration of EVOO phenols to rats co-exposed to aluminum and acrylamide leads to the improvement of their blood lipid profile by reducing TC and increasing HDL-C levels [11]. It has been reported that oxidized LDL-C concentration decreases after a high-phenolic olive oil intake [24]. Moreover, the 3-month consumption of a Med-diet supplemented with virgin olive oil reduces TC and LDL-C and increases HDL-C in high-cardiovascular-risk participants [25].

3.3 Polyphenols and endothelial dysfunction

Endothelial cells are able to synthesize molecules, such as NO and endothelin 1 (ET-1), substances with vasodilator and vasoconstrictor activities, respectively [26, 27]. An imbalance between vasodilating and vasoconstricting molecules induces endothelial dysfunction. At the cellular level, ROS can neutralize the vasodilator NO, inactivate protein tyrosine phosphatases, increase intracellular free calcium concentrations, and act as second messengers within redox-dependent signaling pathways [28]. Endothelial dysfunction, a critical event in the development of hypertension, is controlled by several vasoactive peptides such as angiotensin II and endothelin-1 [29].

The high content of phenolic compounds present in EVOO may slow the atherogenic process by inhibiting oxidative damage and restoring endothelial function. In fact, EVOO phenols decrease endothelial NO synthase phosphorylation, and consequently intracellular NO levels, and increase endothelin-1 synthesis in ECV304 cells incubated with high glucose and fatty acid concentrations [30].

3.4 Polyphenols and hypertension

Hypertension is a serious medical condition characterized by a persistent elevation of the blood pressure in the arteries and reflects a hypersensitivity of the vascular smooth muscle to vasoconstrictor stimuli [31]. It corresponds to a systolic blood pressure (SBP) of 140 mmHg or more and/or to a diastolic blood pressure (DBP) of 90 mmHg or more [32]. It is recognized as one of the strong causes leading to cardiovascular stroke and myocardial infarction [33]. Oxidative stress has been shown to be the fundamental mechanism responsible for hypertension [34]. Other factors, such as inflammation, endothelial dysfunction and vascular remodeling, have been also documented as key contributors to this condition [33]. Reactive oxygen species are involved in the homeostasis of the vascular wall, and particularly in the modulation of the vasomotor system. Superoxide anion can even play the role of a vasoconstrictor agent and it can rapidly react with NO, decreasing the bioavailability of this vasodilator molecule [35]. Enhanced ROS generation and reduced NO levels, in addition to reduced antioxidant status, have been reported in hypertensive humans and animals [36, 37].

On the other hand, several studies have demonstrated that olive oil polyphenols have vasoprotective effects on blood pressure. Moreno-Luna et al. [38] have shown that the daily intake of a polyphenol-rich olive oil diet during 8 weeks is effective in reducing peripheral SBP and DBP in young women with mild hypertension. Recently, Sarapis et al. [39] have reported a decrease in both central and peripheral SBP in healthy adults after the daily consumption of EVOO with high polyphenols content during 3 weeks. The anti-hypertensive effects of olive oil have been mainly attributed to its phenolic compounds. In fact, administration of isolated polyphenols from olive oil, like oleuropein, has shown a positive correlation with the improvement of the hypertensive state [40]. Several mechanisms have been proposed for the blood-pressure lowering effects of olive oil polyphenols. They include, for example, suppression of the oxidative stress and inflammatory processes, enhancement of the endothelial synthesis of NO [38], and modulation of the expression of genes connected to the renin–angiotensin system [41].

3.5 Polyphenols and obesity

During the past few decades, obesity has been considered as a chronic disease resulting from multiple interactions between genetic and lifestyle factors. It is characterized by an increase in the number and size of adipocytes in adipose tissue leading to the development of T2D, CVD and hyperlipidemia [42]. Adiponectin, a major adipocyte -secreted adipokine, is abundantly present in the circulation of healthy humans exerting anti-diabetic and anti-inflammatory activities [43]. In obese individuals, its levels are decreased through mechanisms involving chronic inflammation, oxidative stress and atherosclerosis, which are factors responsible for the development of CVD [43]. Therefore, dietary strategies are effective in modulating adiponectin secretion by the improvement of inflammation-associated adipocyte dysfunction to reduce the risk of obesity-related CVD. Previous studies have suggested that olive polyphenols can inhibit pre-adipocyte differentiation, suppress lipogenesis, induce lipolysis, and regulate adiponectin secretion [44, 45]. HT, at nutritionally relevant concentrations, induces adiponectin down- regulation in human adipocytes through the attenuation of adipogenesis- related genes (JNK-mediated PPARγ) expression [43]. Additionally, Drira et al. [45] have reported that HT and oleuropein at concentrations of 100 and 150 μM and 200 and 300 μM respectively, reduce pre-adipocyte differentiation and lipid accumulation and thus regulate the size of fat cells on 3T3 –L1 cells. It has been proposed that oleuropein may diffuse through the lipid bilayer of the cell membrane and may be absorbed via a glucose transporter [46]. These data indicate that EVOO phenols may play a protective role against excessive fat accumulation by inhibiting the differentiation rate of adipocytes and down-regulation of the adipogenesis-related genes. Therefore, olive oil polyphenols have great effects on the adipogenesis process and can be helpful in the prevention and treatment of obesity-related metabolic and CVDs in humans.

3.6 Polyphenols and diabetes

Diabetes is a chronic metabolic disease which can affect over time the entire body, and particularly the cardiovascular system. Compared to non-diabetic subjects, people suffering from diabetes, notably type 2 diabetes (T2D), have an increased chance of developing CVD [47]. Furthermore, cardiovascular complications represent the main cause of mortality among diabetic patients [48]. These complications can be manifested at the vascular and the cardiac levels. The key pathologic diabetic pathways affecting the vasculature include oxidative stress, alteration of vascular progenitor cells, microvascular dysfunction and impairment in reverse cholesterol transport [49]. Diabetes can also predispose the myocardium to specific structural and functional damages, a condition known as diabetic cardiomyopathy (DCM) in diabetic patients. Several molecular events are known to trigger DCM such as alterations in the metabolism of glucose, ketones, fatty acids and amino acids, impairment of insulin signalling, calcium mishandling, oxidative stress and inflammation [50].

Growing evidence from human and animal researches supports the positive outcome of olive oil consumption, especially EVOO, on diabetes management. Results from the "Prevención con Dieta Mediterránea" (PREDIMED) study have shown a lower incidence of T2D mellitus with an increasing adherence to a Med-diet rich in EVOO in patients at high CVD risk [51]. Also, a Med-diet supplemented with virgin olive oil has been observed to improve glucose metabolism and insulin sensitivity in subjects with T2D [52]. Besides, the daily intake of a polyphenol-rich EVOO during 8 weeks has been demonstrated to significantly reduce the levels of fasting plasma glucose and circulating inflammatory adipokines (cytokines involved in glucose metabolism) in overweight patients with T2D [53]. In an animal study performed on T2D mice, EVOO administration for 24 weeks has been reported to lower fasting glycemia, insulinemia and insulin resistance and to ameliorate β-cells' function [54]. It has been suggested that polyphenols present in EVOO may contribute significantly to its protective role against diabetes [53, 55]. Among them, HT and oleuropein have been demonstrated to display anti-diabetic actions in both *in vivo* and *in vitro* studies [56–58]. Polyphenols might influence glucose metabolism through reducing the digestion and the intestinal absorption of dietary carbohydrates, stimulating insulin secretion, and improving glucose uptake in the tissues by modulating intracellular signaling [59]. Due to their antioxidant properties, these bioactive compounds could also inhibit the formation of advanced glycation endproducts, which results in the protection of pancreatic β-cells against glucotoxicity [60].

4. Conclusions and future perspectives

In summary, multiple beneficial effects on CVD risk factors have been associated with the consumption of Med-diet patterns rich in EVOO. The cardioprotective effects of polyphenols present in olive oil are mediated through the inhibition of atherosclerosis, hypertension, obesity and diabetes, amelioration of the plasma lipid profile and improvement of the endothelial function. The consumption of a Med-diet supplemented with olive oil is therefore recommended, as it could serve as a functional food beyond basic nutrition. Further efforts are needed to elucidate the pharmacokinetics and pharmacodynamics underlying the potential effect of EVOO phenolic compounds and the dose-dependence of their effects in humans.

Author details

Imen Ghorbel[1*], Mariem Chaâbane[1], Naziha Grati Kammoun[2] and Najiba Zeghal[1]

1 Sciences Faculty of Sfax, Animal Physiology Laboratory, University of Sfax, Sfax, Tunisia

2 Laboratory of Resources of the Olive Tree: Characterization, Valorization and Phytosanitary Protection, Technology and Quality Research Unit, Olive Tree Institute, University of Sfax, Sfax, Tunisia

*Address all correspondence to: ghorbel21@gmail.com

References

[1] Visioli F, Bellomo G, Montedoro G, Galli C. Low density lipoprotein oxidation is inhibited in vitro by olive oil constituents. Atherosclerosis. 1995;**117**:25-32

[2] Ghorbel I, Khemakhem M, Boudawara O, Marrekchi R, Jamoussi K, Ben Amar R, et al. Effects of dietary extra virgin olive oil and its fractions on antioxidant status and DNA damage in the heart of rats co-exposed to aluminum and acrylamide. Food & Function. 2015;**9**:3098-3108

[3] Bajoub A, Medina Rodríguez S, Olmo-García L, Ajal EA, Monasterio RP, Hanine H, Fernández-Gutiérrez A, Carrasco-Pancorbo A. In-depth two-year study of phenolic profile variability among olive oils from autochthonous and mediterranean varieties in Morocco, as revealed by a LC-MS chemometric profiling approach. International Journal of Molecular Sciences. 2017;**18**:52

[4] Foscolou A, Critselis E, Panagiotakos D. Olive oil consumption and human health: A narrative review. Maturitas. 2018;**118**:60-66

[5] Rietjens SJ, Bast A, Haenen GRMM. New insights into controversies on the antioxidant potential of the olive oil antioxidant hydroxytyrosol. Journal of Agricultural and Food Chemistry. 2007;**55**:7609-7614

[6] Yubero-Serrano EM, Lopez-Moreno J, Gomez-Delgado F, Lopez-Miranda J. Extra virgin olive oil: More than a healthy fat. European Journal of Clinical Nutrition. 2019;**72**:8-17

[7] Schwingshackl L, Christoph M, Hoffmann G. Effects of olive oil on markers of inflammation and endothelial function—A systematic review and meta-analysis. Nutrients. 2015;**7**:7651-7675

[8] Servili M, Montedoro G. Contribution of phenolic compounds to virgin olive oil quality. European Journal of Lipid Science and Technology. 2002;**104**:602-613

[9] Serreli G, Deiana M. Biological relevance of extra virgin olive oil polyphenols metabolites. Antioxidants. 2018;**7**:170

[10] Kim HS, Quon MJ, Kim JA. New insights into the mechanisms of polyphenols beyond antioxidant properties; lessons from the green tea polyphenol, epigallocatechin 3-gallate. Redox Biology. 2014;**2**:187-195

[11] Ghorbel I, Elwej A, Jamoussi K, Boudawara T, Grati Kamoun N, Zeghal N. Potential protective effects of extra virgin olive oil on the hepatotoxicity induced by co-exposure of adult rats to acrylamide and aluminum. Food & Function. 2015;**4**:1126-1135

[12] Pifarre R. Thrombosis and cardiovascular disease. Medical Clinics of North America. 1998;**82**:511-522

[13] Rajendran P, Rengarajan T, Thangavel J, Nishigaki Y, Sakthisekaran D, Sethi G, et al. The vascular endothelium and human diseases. International Journal of Biological Sciences. 2013;**9**:1057-1069

[14] Panth N, Paudel KR, Parajuli K. Reactive oxygen species: A key hallmark of cardiovascular disease. Advances in Medicine. 2016;**2016**:9152732

[15] Vanhoutte PM, Zhao Y, Xu A, Leung SWS. Thirty years of saying NO. Circulation Research. 2016;**119**:375-396

[16] Lubos E, Handy DE, Loscalzo J. Role of oxidative stress and nitric oxide in atherothrombosis. Frontiers in Bioscience. 2008;**13**:5323-5344

[17] Ruano J, Lopez-Miranda J, de la Torre R, Delgado-Lista J, Fernandez J, Caballero J, et al. Intake of phenol-rich virgin olive oil improves the postprandial prothrombotic profile in hypercholesterolemic patients. The American Journal of Clinical Nutrition. 2007;**86**:341-346

[18] Dell'Agli M, Fagnani R, Mitro N, Scurati S, Masciadri M, Mussoni L, et al. Minor components of olive oil modulate proatherogenic adhesion molecules involved in endothelial activation. Journal of Agricultural and Food Chemistry. 2006;**54**:3259-3264

[19] Cicerale S, Lucas L, Keast R. Biological activities of phenolic compounds present in virgin olive oil. International Journal of Molecular Sciences. 2010;**11**:458-479

[20] Ross R. Atherosclerosis - An inflammatory disease. The New England Journal of Medicine. 1999;**340**:115-126

[21] Members NLC, Myers GL, Christenson RH, Cushman M, Ballantyne CM, Cooper GR, et al. National Academy of Clinical Biochemistry Laboratory Medicine Practice guidelines: Emerging biomarkers for primary prevention of cardiovascular disease. Clinical Chemistry. 2009;**55**:378-384

[22] Zern TL, Fernandez ML. Cardioprotective effects of dietary polyphenols. The Journal of Nutrition. 2005;**135**:2291-2294

[23] Debry PE, Ash A, Neklason DW, Metheral JE. Role of multidrug resistance P- glycoprotein in cholesterol esterification. The Journal of Biological Chemistry. 1997;**272**:1026-1031

[24] Hohmann CD, Cramer H, Michalsen A, Kessler C, Steckhan N, Choi K, et al. Effects of high phenolic olive oil on cardiovascular risk factors: A systematic review and meta-analysis. Phytomedicine. 2015;**22**:631-640

[25] Llorente-Cortes V, Estruch R, Mena MP, Ros E, González MA, Fitó M, et al. Effect of Mediterranean diet on the expression of pro-atherogenic genes in a population at high cardiovascular risk. Atherosclerosis. 2010;**208**:442-450

[26] Ignarro LJ, Buga GM, Wood KS, Byrns RE, Chaudhuri G. Endothelium-derived relaxing factor produced and released from artery and vein is nitric oxide. Proceedings of the National Academy of Sciences of the United States of America. 1987;**84**:9265-9269

[27] Yanagisawa M, Kurihara H, Kimura S, Tomobe Y, Kobayashi M, Mitsui Y, et al. A novel potent vasoconstrictor peptide produced by vascular endothelial cells. Nature. 1988;**332**:411-415

[28] Garcia-Redondo AB, Aguado A, Briones AM, Salaices M. NADPH oxidases and vascular remodeling in cardiovascular diseases. Pharmaceutical Research. 2016;**114**:110-120

[29] Schiffrin EL. Vascular endothelin in hypertension. Vascular Pharmacology. 2005;**43**:19-29

[30] Storniolo CE, Rosello-Catafau J, Pinto X, Mitjavila MT, Moreno JJ. Polyphenol fraction of extra virgin olive oil protects against endothelial dysfunction induced by high glucose and free fatty acids through modulation of nitric oxide

and endothelin-1. Redox Biology. 2014;**2**:971-977

[31] Bohr DF, Webb RC. Vascular smooth muscle membrane in hypertension. Annual Review of Pharmacology and Toxicology. 1988;**28**:389-409

[32] Mirzaei M, Mirzaei M, Bagheri B, Dehghani A. Awareness, treatment, and control of hypertension and related factors in adult Iranian population. BMC Public Health. 2020;**20**:667

[33] Mehmood A, Usman M, Patil P, Zhao L, Wang C. A review on management of cardiovascular diseases by olive polyphenols. Food Science & Nutrition. 2020;**8**:4639-4655

[34] Rodrigo R, González J, Paoletto F. The role of oxidative stress in the pathophysiology of hypertension. Hypertension Research. 2011;**34**:431-440

[35] Baradaran A, Nasri H, Rafieian-Kopaei M. Oxidative stress and hypertension: Possibility of hypertension therapy with antioxidants. Journal of Research in Medical Sciences : The Official Journal of Isfahan University of Medical Sciences. 2014;**19**:358-367

[36] Touyz RM. Reactive oxygen species, vascular oxidative stress, and redox signaling in hypertension: What is the clinical significance? Hypertension. 2004;**44**:248-252

[37] Tanito M, Nakamura H, Kwon YW, Teratani A, Masutani H, Shioji K, et al. Enhanced oxidative stress and impaired thioredoxin expression in spontaneously hypertensive rats. Antioxidants & Redox Signaling. 2004;**6**:89-97

[38] Moreno-Luna R, Muñoz-Hernandez R, Miranda ML, Costa AF, Jimenez-Jimenez L, Vallejo-Vaz AJ, et al. Olive oil polyphenols decrease blood pressure and improve endothelial function in young women with mild hypertension. American Journal of Hypertension. 2012;**25**:1299-1304

[39] Sarapis K, Thomas CJ, Hoskin J, George ES, Marx W, Mayr HL, et al. The effect of high polyphenol extra virgin olive oil on blood pressure and arterial stiffness in healthy australian adults: A randomized, controlled, cross-over study. Nutrients. 2020;**12**:2272

[40] Menezes RCR, Peres KK, Costa-Valle MT, et al. Oral administration of oleuropein and olive leaf extract has cardioprotective effects in rodents: A systematic review. Revista Portuguesa de Cardiologia. 2022;**41**:167-175

[41] Martin-Pelaez S, Castaner O, Konstantinidou V, Subirana I, Munoz-Aguayo D, Blanchart G, et al. Effect of olive oil phenolic compounds on the expression of blood pressure-related genes in healthy individuals. European Journal of Nutrition. 2017;**56**:663-670

[42] Saltiel AR, Kahn CR. Insulin signaling and the regulation of the glucose and lipid metabolism. Nature. 2001;**414**:799-806

[43] Scoditti E, Massaro M, Carluccio MA, Pellegrino M, Wabitsch M, Calabriso N, et al. Additive regulation of adiponectin expression by the mediterranean diet olive oil components oleic acid and hydroxytyrosol in human adipocytes. PLoS One. 2015;**10**:e0128218

[44] Park HS, Kim SH, Kim YS, Ryu SY, Hwang JT, Yang HJ, et al. Luteolin inhibits adipogenic differentiation by regulating PPAR gamma activation. BioFactors. 2009;**35**:373-379

[45] Drira R, Chen S, Sakamoto K. Oleuropein and hydroxytyrosol inhibit

adipocyte differentiation in 3 T3-L1 cells. Life Sciences. 2011;**89**:708-716

[46] Edgecombe SC, Strech GL, Hayball PJ. Oleuropein, an antioxidant polyphenol from olive oil, is poorly absorbed from isolated perfused rat intestine. The Journal of Nutrition. 2000;**130**:2996-3002

[47] Martín-Timón I, Sevillano-Collantes C, Segura-Galindo A, Del Cañizo-Gómez FJ. Type 2 diabetes and cardiovascular disease: Have all risk factors the same strength? World Journal of Diabetes. 2014;**5**:444-470

[48] Dal Canto E, Ceriello A, Rydén L, Ferrini M, Hansen TB, Schnell O, et al. Diabetes as a cardiovascular risk factor: An overview of global trends of macro and micro vascular complications. European Journal of Preventive Cardiology. 2019;**26**:25-32

[49] Kovacic JC, Castellano JM, Farkouh ME, Fuster V. The relationships between cardiovascular disease and diabetes: Focus on pathogenesis. Endocrinology and Metabolism Clinics of North America. 2014;**43**:41-57

[50] Wang L, Cai Y, Jian L, Cheung CW, Liangqing Z. Impact of peroxisome proliferator-activated receptor-α on diabetic cardiomyopathy. Cardiovascular Diabetology. 2021;**20**:2

[51] Salas-Salvadó J, Bulló M, Babio N, Martínez-González MÁ, Ibarrola-Jurado N, Basora J, et al. Reduction in the incidence of type 2 diabetes with the Mediterranean diet: Results of the PREDIMED-Reus nutrition intervention randomized trial. Diabetes Care. 2011;**34**:14-19

[52] Lasa A, Miranda J, Bulló M, Casas R, Salas-Salvadó J, Larretxi I, et al. Comparative effect of two Mediterranean diets versus a low-fat diet on glycaemic control in individuals with type 2 diabetes. European Journal of Clinical Nutrition. 2014;**68**:767-772

[53] Santangelo C, Filesi C, Varì R, Scazzocchio B, Filardi T, Fogliano V, et al. Consumption of extra-virgin olive oil rich in phenolic compounds improves metabolic control in patients with type 2 diabetes mellitus: A possible involvement of reduced levels of circulating visfatin. Journal of Endocrinological Investigation. 2016;**39**:1295-1301

[54] Jurado-Ruiz E, Álvarez-Amor L, Varela LM, et al. Extra virgin olive oil diet intervention improves insulin resistance and islet performance in diet-induced diabetes in mice. Scientific Reports. 2019;**9**:11311

[55] Da Porto A, Brosolo G, Casarsa V, et al. The pivotal role of oleuropein in the anti-diabetic action of the Mediterranean diet: A concise review. Pharmaceutics. 2021;**14**:40

[56] Jemai H, El Feki A, Sayadi S. Antidiabetic and antioxidant effects of hydroxytyrosol and oleuropein from olive leaves in alloxan-diabetic rats. Journal of Agricultural and Food Chemistry. 2009;**57**:8798-8804

[57] Wu L, Velander P, Liu D, Xu B. Olive component oleuropein promotes β-cell insulin secretion and protects β-cells from amylin amyloid-induced cytotoxicity. Biochemistry. 2017;**56**:5035-5039

[58] Vlavcheski F, Young M, Tsiani E. Antidiabetic effects of hydroxytyrosol: In vitro and in vivo evidence. Antioxidants. 2019;**8**:188

[59] Alkhatib A, Tsang C, Tuomilehto J. Olive oil nutraceuticals in the prevention and management of diabetes: From

molecules to lifestyle. International Journal of Molecular Sciences. 2018;**19**:2024

[60] Xiao JB, Högger P. Dietary polyphenols and type 2 diabetes: Current insights and future perspectives. Current Medicinal Chemistry. 2015;**22**:23-38

Section 3

Strategies for Nutritional Security

Chapter 5

Biofortification of Rice, An Impactful Strategy for Nutritional Security: Current Perspectives and Future Prospect

Kuntal Das, Priyabrata Roy and Raj Kumar Singh Tiwari

Abstract

Globally, especially in the developing world, an estimated 20,000 million people are affected by micronutrient deficiency, generally named "hidden hunger". Crop biofortification is an impactful strategy in addressing nutritional security as well as providing a cost-saving, sustainable means by uplifting health and well-being to communities with deprived access to diversified foods and interventions regarding the micronutrient supply. Considering the global concerns about micronutrient deficiency, research organizations have initiated studies on ensuring the bioavailability of micronutrients in staple food crops. Mitigating hidden hunger with the biofortification of rice surely can be a beneficial strategy for people who consumes rice as a staple food. Significant enhancement in iron and zinc levels, as well as with other essential minerals and vitamins is achieved in rice biofortification by various approaches. Adoption of biofortified rice varieties in targeted countries would significantly increase daily micronutrient intake and help to holistically alleviate malnutrition in human populations. This review articulates the status and perspective of rice biofortification as well as summarizes dissemination and adoption along with trends in consumer acceptance. With a positive trend, attention should now need shift to an action-based agenda and robust policy directives for scaling up rice biofortification in improving nutritional security for humans.

Keywords: rice, biofortification, malnutrition, micronutrient, hidden hunger, adoption

1. Introduction

For thousands of years, rice has remained a significant part of the human diet. Rice was cultivated and consumed up to 10,000 years ago, according to historical evidence, and it is still the world's most significant and accepted meal for humans, sustaining more people over a longer period than any other crop. Rice will continue to be a vital staple meal for billions of people in the future, making it one of the most crucial agricultural commodities in the world and is immensely linked with food security, economic growth, employment, culture, and regional peace of a nation. For half of the global population, represented by more than 3 billion people worldwide, rice has been an important crop for many countries. Rice not only meets the basic food demands but also contributes significantly to the economic growth of rice-growing countries through exports. Globally rice crop is estimated to cover 164.7 million acres [1]. Asia accounts for 90–92% of total rice acreage and is a major producer and consumer of rice [2]. To feed the world's rising population, rice output has increased significantly, from 220 million tons in the pre-green revolution era to 729 million tons in 2017. Rice accounts for around 20% of per capita energy and 13% of the protein consumed by humans worldwide and contributes much more dietary energy and protein than 29.3 dietary energy and 29.1% dietary protein in many poor countries [3].

The health risks associated with micronutrient insufficiency in humans have become the main obstacle to meeting the Sustainable Development Goals (SDGs) set for 2035, which include reducing hunger and poverty, improving maternal health, and lowering child mortality. Micronutrients, though at trace levels are detrimental to the human body for general healthy growth and development. Micronutrient shortage has been associated with higher sickness and death rates, lower income, and detrimental impacts on infant and child growth, subsequent physical and mental development, and learning. The deficiency of iron and zinc is one of humanity's most common scenarios, affecting 2 billion people globally and resulting in more than 0.8 million fatalities every year [4]. Micronutrient deficiencies are prominently detected in nearly two-thirds of all child mortality attributable to dietary inadequacies [5]. Hidden hunger can be decreased by adopting both direct (nutrition-specific) and indirect (nutrition-sensitive) techniques [6]. Direct treatments that target consumption habits include dietary diversification, vitamin supplementation, modifying food preferences, and fortification. Crop biofortification and addressing the underlying causes of malnutrition are examples of nutrition-sensitive therapy.

Biofortification is the process of increasing critical nutrient constituents and bioavailability in crops during the growth of plants by genetics and agronomic mechanisms [7]. In genetic biofortification, either traditional breeding or genetic engineering is applied [8]. Agronomic biofortification can be accomplished through the application of micronutrient fertilizers to the soil and/or foliar applications made directly to the crop's leaves. Rice, wheat, corn, sorghum, millet sweet potatoes, and legumes are the primary targets of biofortification because they cover the majority of human diets worldwide, particularly for populations at risk of nutritional deficiencies having limited access to diversified diets, fortified foods, and marketed food supplements [9]. Although biofortification is universally accepted to be useful and is being implemented more effectively, the addition of only one nutrient per crop, either iron, zinc, or provitamin, remains a constraint. The breeding and the release process of the first wave of biofortified cultivars had taken 8–10 years. There are a few cases where the target crop species have enough genetic variation to add a second nutrient through traditional breeding methods, but this is expected to take several years.

There are numerous approaches to alleviating malnutrition induced by a lack of nutritional diversity. To assure micronutrient adequacy in populations, industrial fortification (*e.g.,* iodine to salt, vitamins A and D to margarine, fluoride to toothpaste, and folic acid to flour) has been employed successfully. Supplementation is the distribution and ingestion of micronutrient-containing tablets, syrup, or capsules and has been used in both developed and developing countries. Even if micronutrients are offered free to customers, fortification, and supplementation both necessitate some level of manufacturing and/or delivery infrastructure, as well as the purchase of micronutrients. As a result, the human population who are marginalized and in need of micronutrients in their diets may be disadvantaged. Biofortification is an effective method for increasing micronutrient levels in widely consumed food crops such as rice. Furthermore, it is a practical and sustainable means of mitigating deficiencies related to micronutrients in people who primarily eat rice and have limited access to a range of foods or markets, and lack access to high-quality medical care [10]. Biofortification of staple crops, such as rice, is a promising technique for improving human health by boosting the nutrient density of meals. The readiness of consumers and farmers to adopt and use new biofortified crop varieties influences the technique's viability. HarvestPlus is primarily focused on the release and distribution of biofortified varieties in Bangladesh, Indonesia, and India. In Asia, breeding programs at the International Rice Research Institute (IRRI), Bangladesh Rice Research Institute (BRRI), Indonesian Center for Rice Research (ICRR), and India's National Agricultural Research System (NARS) have produced germplasm from early to late developmental stages, as well as elite lines and released a few varieties. Additionally, zinc-rich breeding pipelines aimed at Latin America were developed at the International Center for Tropical Agriculture (CIAT). HarvestPlus focuses on inbred varieties rather than hybrids because hybrids are not yet widely accepted outside of China. The crop's availability and knowledge of its health advantages are two of the most critical factors for the acceptance and adoption of biofortified crops. Much of the research reviewed here reveal that biofortified crops were not readily available to the general people, and acceptance and adoption remained questionable. Many biofortified rice products have already completed the development phase, which should result in additional evidence of the substitution of current cultivars with biofortified types and the changes in consumer diets.

The purpose of this chapter is to understand the relevance of addressing micronutrient deficiencies as well as other types of nutritional inadequacies to minimize hidden hunger in all its manifestations, which remains one of the most difficult challenges in public health. The chapter also elucidates the likely causes and factors of hidden hunger, reviewing its global prevalence, and explores current strategies to mitigate it through rice biofortification. The authors hope that this chapter, along with our collective efforts, will provide a suitable platform for constructive dialog among scientists, researchers, entrepreneurs, policymakers, and growers to reduce the burgeoning issues of malnutrition with holistic information, approaches, and means as well as take a serious step in developing biofortified rice with their release and promotion for augmented adoption.

2. Malnutrition: the hidden hunger

Human health and well-being are dependent on proper nutrition. Every person on this planet has the right to safe, sufficient, and nutritious food, as well as the right to be free from all forms of food insecurity. However, one out of every three individuals worldwide suffers from some form of malnutrition, such as undernutrition, micronutrient deficiency, being overweight, or obesity, which leads to a variety of clinical illnesses. If current trends continue, the situation will deteriorate since malnutrition is projected to affect one out of every two people worldwide [11]. High levels of malnutrition are likely to persist unless humans have access to inexpensive healthcare facilities, safe drinking water and sanitization, affordable agricultural inputs, accessible technical help, education, employment, and social safety programs [11]. Combating hunger in all its manifestations is one of the most important concerns confronting many countries nowadays. The United Nations Decade of Action on Nutrition (2016–2025) reached its halfway point. However, the proportion of persons suffering from malnutrition has risen since 2015. One of the 17 SDGs is to eliminate hunger by 2030, and the UN Food Systems Summit and Nutrition for Growth Summit in 2021 emphasized a renewed emphasis on global nutritional research.

The term hidden hunger refers to the scenario of certain micronutrient deficiencies in the absence of diverse energy and nutrient rice diet. Hidden hunger is estimated to afflict over two billion people globally, particularly in low- and middle-income countries, where people rely on low-cost staples that are nutrition deficient, and their nutritious food options are limited due to lack of access and poverty. A long-term, cost-effective solution to eliminating hidden hunger is the need of the hour and must be able to reach the most isolated and neglected places. A system approach involving all aspects of the food value chain is essential to enable safe and sustainable food security that is resilient to external volatile market shocks. Even while the most severe occurrence of hidden hunger is experienced in developing countries, dietary deficiencies can affect anyone, at any age, and from any ethnic background around the world [12]. This remains one of the most significant impediments to socioeconomic advancement, leading to a vicious cycle of hunger, poverty, and underdevelopment. Although the impoverished world bears a greater proportion of the burden of hidden hunger, micronutrient inadequacy, particularly iodine and iron deficiency are highly ubiquitous around the world (**Figure 1**) [13]. Among micronutrient deficits, it is evident from **Figure 1** that vitamin A deficiency is of the highest concern for children below 5 years of age globally (~33%), where the same as the continent-specific situation has been highest in Africa and lowest in Oceania. This is followed by iodine deficiency, which is ~29% globally and the same as the continent-specific situation been highest in Europe and lowest in Oceania. Vitamin A deficiency is highest in pregnant women in Asia, whereas iron deficiency in pregnant women is highest in Africa.

Micronutrient deficiency has long-term consequences for health, mental function, and efficiency, resulting in enormous social and public expenditures, lower working capacity due to high sickness and disability rates, and severe health risks. Low-income, resource-poor communities, socially excluded groups, and economically disenfranchised food-insecure households are usually among the most nutritionally challenged.

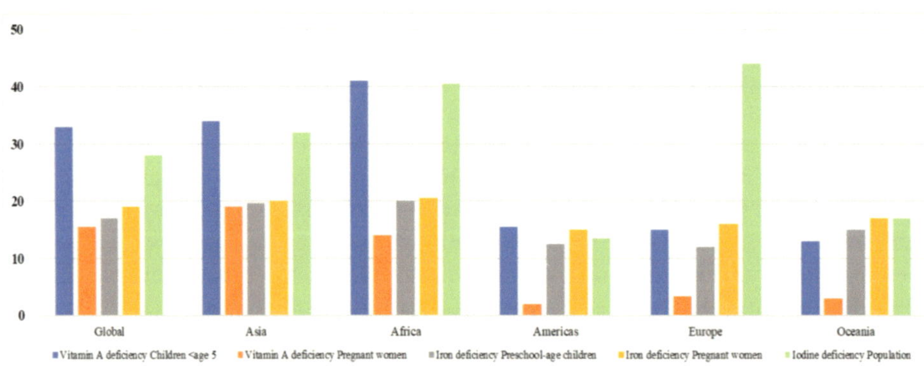

Figure 1.
Global population (in percentage) with major micronutrient deficiencies across continents. X-axis shows the global and continents, affected population in percentage in Y-axis as bars. Source: Ref. [13].

2.1 Goal of achieving zero hunger

One of the UN's SDGs is to end hunger by attaining food security and improved nutrition, as well as supporting sustainable agriculture. In the context of this goal of zero hunger, several internationally agreed-upon targets have been defined, all of which must be met by 2030. Within this framework, performance objectives have been devised to allow different nations to monitor their progress, such as a decrease in the prevalence of stunting and malnutrition. Globally, little progress has been made to mitigate and minimize the proportion of children under the age of five suffering from severe malnutrition, which decreased from 23.1% in 2015 to 21.3% in 2019 [14]. Even while stunting has grown less widespread in recent years, 14 million children under the age of five were still affected in 2019, with Asia and Africa accounting for three-quarters of those affected. In terms of childhood obesity, 38 million children under the age of five were overweight in 2019 [15], and the figure is steadily rising in various nations. Asia was home to over half of all obese children under the age of five in 2019. Despite progress in combating malnutrition, the United Nations has expressed that the world is not on track to achieving hunger-free status by 2030.

2.2 Drive for diet diversification

Dietary diversity is an evaluation of an individual's consumption of various foods from assorted food groups over a certain period. Analyzing dietary diversity patterns is an important tool in developing a strategic work plan to combat hidden hunger, since a diverse diet is less likely to be lacking in micronutrient supplies. Questionnaire-based approaches to assessing food diversity at the population level have been developed, which offers an advantage in determining nutrient consumption in a streamlined approach by acquiring data that does not rely on thorough, time-consuming food studies or highly competent enumerators.

2.3 Drive for nutrient supplementation

Nutrient supplementation can give a direct solution when nutritional deficiencies can be detected. Systematic reviews of the kinds of literature show that supplementation programs can increase micronutrient levels. Folate and iron supplements given to women of reproductive phases around the world have helped in improving anemia and pregnancy outcomes. Supplementation to cure hidden hunger at the community level is a difficult task and is dependent on public involvement since it is expensive and depends on the ability to reach those most vulnerable populations. Supplementation can help in the short term, but it will not solve the long-term problem of a nutrient-deficient diet.

2.4 Food fortification

The addition of nutrients to foods during the processing just before consumption is referred to as food fortification. One of the most successful fortification methods employed globally has been the fortification of iodine to edible salts. Iodine deficiency has substantial adverse health effects, which are associated with its crucial role in the synthesis of thyroid hormone causing stunted growth and limited cognitive development in humans. Many countries mandate iodine fortification of salts, with United Nations International Childers's Emergency Fund (UNICEF) reporting 86%

household approval worldwide [16]. The efficiency of a comprehensive fortification strategy depends on the successful supply and accessibility of fortified products, ensuring their availability in targeted locations. Furthermore, the fortifying system must be properly developed and monitored for quality management and safety, with at least regional-level supervision with adequate investment. As a result, food fortification favors metropolitan areas with better infrastructure for distributing fortified products than rural areas and higher socioeconomic status and health-related awareness.

2.5 Global perspective of hidden hunger

More than 2 billion people worldwide experience hidden hunger, out of 805 million people who do not have enough calories to eat [17]. Several variables contribute to this difficulty, as indicated briefly in **Figure 2**.

The South Asian subcontinent and a vast area of Africa, south of the Sahara, where hidden hunger is prevalent. Frequencies are quite low in Latin America and the Caribbean, where diets rely less on a single crop and are more influenced by significant usage of vitamin supplementation, education initiatives, and basic health care [18]. While malnutrition is more widespread in developing countries, iron, and iodine deficits are also common in developed countries. The worldwide malnutrition

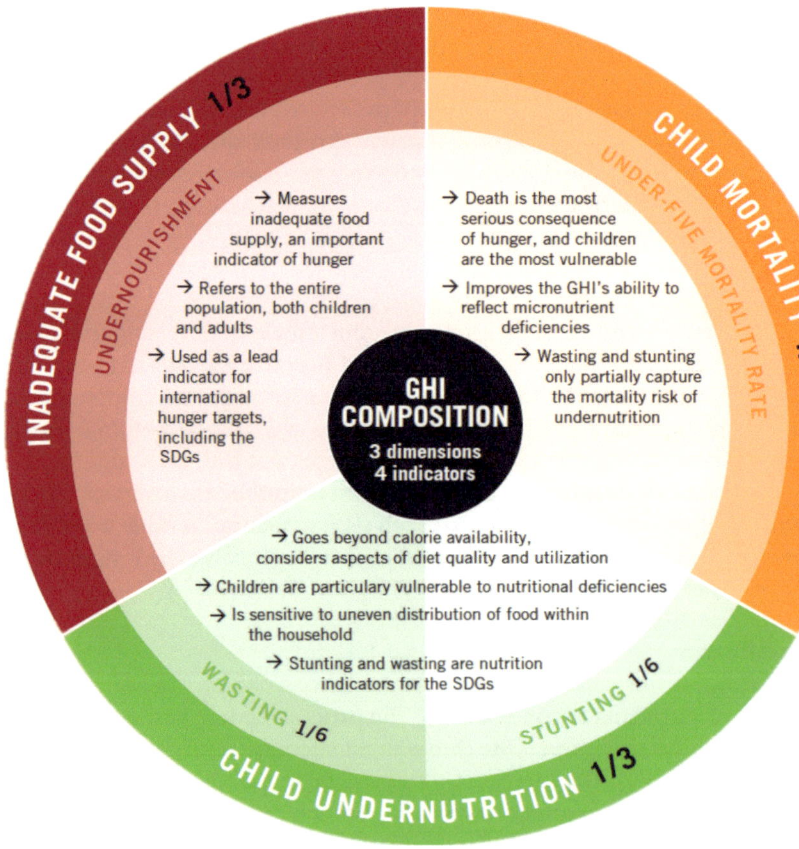

Figure 2.
A brief outline of the composition of the Global Hunger Index. Source: Ref. [13].

problem is becoming more complex. Developing countries are shifting away from traditional diets and inclining to processed meals, calorie-dense diets, and beverages that are low in micronutrients and contribute to obesity and chronic diseases associated with it. Micronutrient deficiencies are estimated to account for 1.1 million of the 3.1 million child deaths caused by malnutrition every year [19]. Vitamin A and zinc deficiency harmed children's health and survival by weakening the immune system. Zinc deficiency both inhibits and causes stunted growth in youngsters. Iodine and iron deficiency inhibit youngsters from reaching their full physical and intellectual potential [20]. The eating habits of women before conception and throughout pregnancy have long-term effects on the growth and development of the fetus. Iodine deficiency causes brain damage in about 18 million infants each year. Severe anemia is the potential cause of the deaths of 50,000 women giving birth each year. Furthermore, iron deficiency causes low energy levels in 40% of women in underdeveloped nations [21]. Typically, efforts to reduce hidden hunger and improve nutrition performance target women, babies, and children. Interventions aimed at these individuals have a high rate of return because they improve later-life health, nutrition, and cognition [22]. The severity of most micronutrient deficits is difficult to communicate. There is a scarcity of data on the prevalence of certain micronutrient deficits. Scientists have not agreed on the usually recommended intakes for several of the 19 micronutrients that directly influence immune function, and physical and mental development [23]. Furthermore, it is unknown how different micronutrient intakes, and their benefits connect to one another. There are numerous significant micronutrients for which prevalence data are absent because appropriate biomarkers for nutritional insufficiency have yet to be discovered. If these data gaps persist, determining the full degree of hidden hunger will be challenging.

When all other measures fail to alleviate hidden hunger, biofortification is likely the only rationally viable choice. It provides a different and more cost-effective approach to increasing nutritional value and status in vulnerable populations. Once the biofortified variety is developed, the seed can be widely distributed and replicated by farmers as farm-saved seeds year after year, so boosting informal seed systems. Following the initial investment in breeding, ongoing costs are cheap, though help may be necessary to optimize fertilizer use to maximize the crop's nutritional content potential. There is also an urgent and rigorous need to investigate the source of crop genotypes high in nutritional value, such as traditional landraces, and local variants, to generate biofortified products.

3. Rice with ethno-nutritional value

Neolithic people began domesticating numerous plants and animals around 12,000 years ago. This sparked the agricultural revolution, which resulted in the development of hundreds of animal breeds and crop landraces, as well as new animal and plant species [24–26]. Around 12,000 and 10,000 years ago in China (*O. sativa* ssp. *japonica*) and India (*O. indica* ssp. *indica*), respectively, rice is developed from the primordial *Oryza rufipogon*, through careful selection of domesticated rice (*Oryza sativa* L.) [27, 28]. Over millennia, local farmers have developed and cultivated hundreds of different rice landraces through painstaking selection and breeding trials. Crop genetic variety is the foundation for adaptability to environmental conditions, such as drought, seasonal flooding, salinity, and crop pest and disease resistance [29, 30]. Agricultural liberalization and industrialization processes, which homogenize the genetic basis, lessen the complexity of agroecosystems, and are associated with increased crop yields, have, nevertheless, depleted the rich reservoirs of natural crop diversity since the green revolution began in the late 1960s [30]. This has damaged farmers' ability to control their food supply, resulting in local and national food insecurity [31]. For example, in India, which is a major rice-growing country, more than 90% of local rice landraces disappeared from agricultural areas between 1970 and 2000 [31]. The extinction of traditional rice genotypes threatens local culinary ethnicities as well as food security, which has disastrous consequences. Farmers who are willing to grow a few heirloom rice varieties despite high market prices are themselves uncommon species, as traditional cultural values associated with local landraces have mostly disappeared within sophisticated farming communities. Folk rice landraces are rapidly disappearing from farmer fields due to a lack of both cultural and economic motivation.

3.1 Indigenous knowledge systems and folk rice landraces

Aside from its agronomic benefits, Rice has a different cultural significance among major nations. Traditional farmers developed, nurtured, and maintained several folk rice varieties that were specifically tailored to the soil and climate of a specific region. Prior to the introduction of modern agriculture at the request of statutory authorities and the seed industry, most marginal farmers used to recollect their specific agronomic features and cultural purposes. Each landrace has its own unique climate, soil conditions, and adaptability. Local landraces are the ideal resource for developing superior cultivars since they contain a diverse set of genes for pest and disease resistance, as well as various nutritional attributes. Many farmer landraces can withstand situations such as severe rain, late rain, insufficient rain, prolonged flooding, and soil salinity that are sometimes missing in modern high-yielding cultivars [30]. Local acceptability is determined by aroma and amylose levels, which also influence how sticky cooked rice is. Several landraces are preferred for making beaten rice, puffed rice, rice pudding, and other delicacies. Esthetic preference is another aspect in the selection and breeding of distinct landraces with colors, such as red, black, purple, and gold for the awn and pericarp, as well as brown, purple, and black for the hull [30].

Many traditional rice varieties have different nutritional properties and medical purposes. In India, Laicha rice from Chhattisgarh and Nyavara rice from Kerala are two examples of medicinal rice used to treat peptic ulcers and chronic gastritis in India. Nyavara has traditionally been used to alleviate neurotic issues. Kabiraj-sal is recommended as a meal for recovering patients' traditional medicine because it includes nutritional properties that improve overall wellness. Garib-sal is the only rice type known to contain silver in its grains, and it is utilized in traditional medicine to cure gastroenteric disorders [32]. The considerable amount of silver on the grains' pericarp of Garib-sal, presumably promotes dangerous intestinal bacteria [32]. One of the South Indian versions, Mappillai samba, has antidiabetic and anticancer properties, as well as steroidal bioactive compounds and antioxidants [33]. Patients suffering from dysentery in Bihar and Jharkhand are given a paste made from the Karanga rice variety. In Assam, patients with jaundice are treated with starchy water from the Bora type of traditional rice [34].

Numerous laboratory studies have already shown that rice and its byproducts have anticancer characteristics and can be used to treat illnesses, such as diabetes, kidney problems, and excessive cholesterol. Although rice is commonly considered a starchy food, it also contains a significant amount of proteins, fatty acids, fiber, many minerals, and vitamins required for normal metabolic functioning [35]. Scientific evidence supports some of rice's medical properties [36, 37]. Rice has antioxidant properties that can prevent cancer, and some traditional rice varieties with a low glycemic index can significantly check blood glucose levels and lower the risk of developing diabetes [38]. According to research, colored rice, such as traditional red and black rice, outperforms high-yielding types in terms of numerous nutritional and medicinal properties [39]. Rakktashali red rice was mentioned in ancient Ayurvedic writings as both food and medicine [40]. Ayurvedic practices typically employ Kerala's well-known Nayavara rice as a body-enhancing material to combat pollutants and slow aging [41]. The pigmented black and red kinds are higher in minerals and polyphenols, which can fortify cells. Basmati rice, which is commonly used in weight-loss programs, has a low glycemic index [42]. Rice is a terrific diet for giving our bodies micronutrients, rejecting toxic metabolites, strengthening, rejuvenating, and revitalizing the body, managing blood pressure, and preventing skin disorders and premature aging due to its antioxidant characteristics [43]. Thousands of traditional rice landraces, which are only available to marginal farmers and conservationists, should be scientifically validated for their healing properties. To maintain these landraces, public awareness campaigns that compete with the existing market of high-yielding cultivars must be created.

4. Rice biofortification for nutritional security

Malnutrition affects over two billion people worldwide, while 815 million people are undernourished. Biofortification is a food-based technique for combating malnutrition by bringing nutrient-dense crops to the doorsteps of poor and needy populations [7]. Biofortification can increase the content of micronutrients in food crops. Biofortified crop types can be offered to populations that do not have access to or cannot afford diversified diets. Biofortification was listed as one of the most significant interventions to eliminate micronutrient deficiencies in low- and middle-income countries in both the 2008 Copenhagen Consensus and the 2013 Lancet series on maternal and child malnutrition. It is also one of the most cost-effective treatments for micronutrient deficiencies, with a 17-dollar return on investment (Copenhagen Consensus). The biofortification technique was initially implemented in the mid-1990s. Biofortification has now received a much bigger financial commitment thanks to the HarvestPlus initiative, which began in 2003 and has financed research projects and biofortification implementation programs all around the world. HarvestPlus is not the only organization that uses biofortification; it is also engaged in regional plant breeding efforts and government programs.

More than half of the world's population derives their energy from rice, a popular staple grain, particularly in Asia that supplies up to 70% of its daily calories. Addressing hidden hunger by rice biofortification may be a sustainable alternative method for those who predominantly consume rice and have limited access to other nutrients. The biofortification procedure successfully raised the number of provitamins and essential minerals in rice grain. Milled rice loses several vital elements such as thiamin and vitamin B due to processing. Furthermore, the grinding and polishing processes destroy 67% of vitamin B3, 80% of vitamin B1, 90% of vitamin B6, 50% of the manganese and phosphorus, 60% of the iron, and all the dietary fiber and important fatty acids. While the consumers prefer white rice grains that are lighter, softer, more easily digestible, and have better eating and cooking qualities, the nutritional quality is compromised when rice is milled and polished due to the loss of the bran layer, the sub aleurone, the embryo, and a small portion of the endosperm [44–47]. Even though education and awareness have improved brown rice consumption, the great majority of rice consumers still choose white polished rice. Researchers should consider developing nutritionally enhanced rice varieties via biofortification (endosperm specific) that can retain nutrients even after processing and polishing. The newly produced biofortified crop varieties, in addition to being an essential source of income for the poor, are also crucial in terms of nutritional security.

5. Biofortified rice: a food-based product to tackle malnutrition

The human body needs nutrition through micronutrients for proper growth and development and to maintain good health [48, 49]. However, shortages of these minerals, as well as the related health risks, are frequent among humans of all ages [50]. Micronutrient malnutrition affects an estimated one-third of the global population because of their significant reliance on cereal staples for daily energy demands and lack of varied diets for nutrient supplementation [51]. Rice biofortification is a novel, promising, cost-effective, and long-term strategy for providing micronutrients to people who do not have access to a varied diet or other micronutrient-based remedies. Unfortunately, our major food crops lack the micronutrients required for normal human development. Until now, our agricultural system has been designed primarily to improve grain yield and crop productivity, with little emphasis on improving human health. However, in the modern era, agriculture is transitioning away from

Biofortified nutrients	Context of research	Publications
Beta-carotene Phytoene (precursor of beta-carotene)	Golden rice and its nutritional value; beta-carotene metabolism; genetic engineering provitamin	[56–59]
Folate (vitamin B9)	Folate fortification and stability; metabolic engineering	[60, 61]
Iron	Nicotianamine aminotransferase genes; transgenic; multigene introduction; ferritin gene; endosperm biofortification	[62–70]
Phytic acid	Iron bioavailability and dietary reference values	[71]
Zinc	Over-expression of OsIRT1; involvement of genes for phytosiderophore synthesis	[72, 73]
High amino acid and protein content	Accumulation of glycinin with the glutelins; dihydrodipicolinate synthase gene; tryptophan accumulation; over-expression of aspartate aminotransferase genes	[63, 74–78]
Alpha-linolenic acid	Microsomal omega-3 fatty acid desaturase gene	[79]
Flavonoids and antioxidants	Flavonoids synthesis in the endosperm; transgenic	[80, 81]
Resistant starch	Amylose level control; antisense waxy gene; physicochemical properties	[82–84]
Human lactoferrin	Expression of human lactoferrin for the application in infant formula	[85]

Table 1.
Research publications on rice biofortification through the transgenic approach.

Biofortified nutrients	Context of research	Publications
Iron	Foliar application; iron fertilizers; grain accumulation; and grain nutritional quality	[86–89]
Zinc	Foliar application at different growth stages; impact on seedling vigor; yield; with pesticides; zinc sulfate; and zinc oxide coatings	[86, 88, 90–94]
Se	Foliar application as fertilizers; sodium selenate; effects on human serum selenium levels; brown rice; selenate-enriched urea granules; antioxidant activity	[86, 95–98]

Table 2.
Research publications on rice biofortification through the agronomic approach.

Variety name	Duration (Days)	Yield (t/ha)	Grain type	Institute, Country	Release Year	Biofortified nutrient
CR Dhan 310	125	4.5	Medium Slender	NRRI, Cuttack, India	2016	Protein (10.3%)
CR Dhan 311 (Mukul)	120–125	4.6	Long Bold	NRRI, Cuttack, India	2018	Protein (10.1%) and Zinc (20.1 ppm)
Bauna Kalanamak 101	135	3.5–4.0	Medium Slender	PRDF, Gorakhpur, India	2016	Zinc (18.9), Fe (4.6 ppm)
Bauna Kalanamak 102	135	4.5	Medium Slender	PRDF, Gorakhpur, India	2016	Zinc (20.75 ppm) and Fe (4.4 ppm)
Binadhan 20	125–130	4.5–7.0		Bangladesh Institute of Nuclear Agriculture (BINA), Bangladesh	2017	Zinc (26.5 ppm), Fe (20–31 ppm)
BRRI Dhan 100	148	7.7	Slender	Bangladesh Rice Research Institute (BRRI), Bangladesh	2020	Zinc (25.6 ppm)
BRRI Dhan 62	100–105	3.5–4.5	Slender	Bangladesh Rice Research Institute (BRRI), Bangladesh	2013	Zinc (19 ppm), Protein (9%)
BRRI Dhan 64	88–100	6.0	Medium Slender	Bangladesh Rice Research Institute (BRRI), Bangladesh	2014	Zinc (23.1 ppm), Fe (36.6 ppm)
BRRI Dhan 72	125–130	5.7	Long bold	Bangladesh Rice Research Institute (BRRI), Bangladesh	2015	Zinc (22.8 ppm), Protein (8.9%)
BRRI Dhan 84	140–145	6.0–6.5	Medium Slender	Bangladesh Rice Research Institute (BRRI)	2017	Zinc (27.6 ppm)

Variety name	Duration (Days)	Yield (t/ha)	Grain type	Institute, Country	Release Year	Biofortified nutrient
Chhattisgarh Zinc Rice 1	112	4.2	Long Slender	IGKV, Raipur, India	2016	Zinc (21.7 ppm)
Chhattisgarh Zinc Rice 2	120–125	4.5	Short Slender	IGKV, Raipur, India	2019	Zinc (>24 ppm)
CR Dhan 315	130	5.0	Medium Slender	NRRI, Cuttack, India	2020	Zinc (24.9 ppm)
CR Dhan 411	140	5.0–6.0	Medium Slender	NRRI, Cuttack, India	2021	Protein (10%)
DRR Dhan 45	130	5.0	Long Slender	IIRR, Hyderabad, India	2016	Zinc (22.6 ppm)
DRR Dhan 48	135–140	5.2	Medium Slender	IIRR, Hyderabad, India	2018	Zinc (24 ppm)
DRR Dhan 49	125–130	5.0–5.5	MS	DRR, Hyderabad, India	2018	Zinc (25.2 ppm
GNR 4	130–135	4.0–5.0	Long Slender	Navsari Agricultural University, Navsari, India	2016	Fe (50 ppm)
Kalanamak Kiran	135	5.0	Medium Slender	Participatory Rural Development Foundation (PRDF), Gorakhpur, India	2019	Protein (10.4%), Zinc, Fe
Ratnagiri 7	122–125	4.5	Short Bold	Agricultural Research Station, Shirgaon, Ratnagiri, India	2019	Zinc (24.25 ppm), Fe (7.9 ppm)
Swarna Shakti Dhan	115–120	4.5–5.0	SB	ICAR-RCER, Patna, India	2020	Zinc (23.5 ppm), Fe (15.1 ppm)
Swarna Sukha Dhan	110–115	3.5–4.0	MS	ICAR-RCER, Patna, India	2021	Zinc (23.1)
Zinco Rice MS	125–130	5.8	MS	IGKV, Raipur, India	2018	Zinc (27.4 ppm)

Table 3.
Details of rice biofortified varieties developed through the breeding approach in South Asia.

high-yielding food crops and toward nutrient-rich food crops, notably cereals, to help combat "hidden hunger" or "micronutrient malnutrition". This is particularly noticeable in emerging nations, where diets are dominated by micronutrients-deficient main food crops such as rice [52].

The development of nutritionally enhanced, high-yielding biofortified crops is one of the primary priorities of organizations such as the World Health Organization (WHO) and the Consultative Group on International Agricultural Research (CGIAR) [53]. Nutritional goals for biofortification include greater mineral content, better vitamin content, increased essential amino acid levels, improved fatty acid composition,

DOI: http://dx.doi.org/10.5772/intechopen.110460

and increased antioxidant levels in crops [54]. Crop plant biofortification can provide enough calories to meet energy needs while also delivering all the essential nutrients needed to maintain excellent human health. Furthermore, biofortified crops consumed by the world's impoverished can significantly improve the well-being of the population of a specific geographic location [55]. Transgenic (**Table 1**), agronomic (**Table 2**), and breeding procedures (**Table 3**) are the three major the techniques for biofortification of essential micronutrients in agricultural plants. A few updates on previous attempts by researchers / scientific workers and the outcomes of these three approaches are depicted below.

6. Dissemination and adoption trends of biofortified rice varieties

The widespread adoption of biofortified rice cultivars is reliant on the availability of appropriate varietal seeds, timely certification, and premium market pricing. As a result, efforts must be made to make these types of varietal seeds available on the market and to ensure premium pricing to entice producers with a value proposition. It is critical to recognize that biofortified crops require far more than a strong marketing push. Acceptability and augmented adoption of biofortified cultivars required significant policy-level interventions in the form of cost subsidies. HarvestPlus-led delivery efforts require around 9.7 million agricultural households to produce biofortified food in 2020, which will be consumed by 48.5 million people worldwide [99]. The global market for biofortification was estimated to be valued at approximately US $72 million in 2017 and is expected to grow to US $117 million over the next several years, rising at an 8.6% CAGR (Compound Annual Growth Rate). Rising consumer demand for high-nutritional-value foods, as well as advances in agricultural technology, are driving this increase.

The willingness of consumers and farmers to accept newly produced nutrient-rich seeds will be a critical success factor for biofortification [9]. Producers' decisions about using biofortified crops will be impacted by yield, disease resistance, drought tolerance, and marketability. Consumer perceptions of biofortified varieties based on sensory features can considerably influence their uptake. A separate technique can be used to access the components that determine nutrient-rich varietal adoption (reflection of intention, initial decision, or action in testing an innovation) and acceptance (reflection of perception among the producers and consumers that innovation is fit for purpose) [100]. Preference testing and sensory studies reveal information on sensory features that influence consumer acceptability (**Table 4**).

Cross-sectional questionnaire surveys reveal attitudes, impediments, and factors that aid or hinder consumers' or producers' adoption of biofortified cultivars. Effective experiments with frequent contrast intensities and less severe treatments are required to evaluate whether biofortified crops are acceptable and are adopted over a specific period. A comparative viewpoint for the acceptability of biofortified varieties against non-biofortified varieties should be mapped, indicating the need for a potential marketing and premium proposition when introducing these cultivars to the targeted territory [105].

Consumer acceptability of biofortified crops varies widely depending on crop type, locality, and consumer characteristics such as age, gender, socioeconomic level, and whether they prefer or dislike biofortified meals (**Table 5**).

Biofortified crops appear to be sensory acceptable to both rural and urban cultures when cooked using traditional methods or as an ingredient in nontraditional food items. The availability of biofortified varieties in the market and thorough knowledge

Publication	Country	Conclusion
Study on gender-specific acceptability of Zinc fortified rice within China [101].	China	Biofortified rice is the least chosen. Acceptance can be improved when rice is cultivated locally, the government encourages it, and the rice kernels are large.
Study on sensory evaluation of rice in Nicaragua [102].	Nicaragua	The study population did not readily accept Azucena.
Study on sensory evaluation of biofortified rice in Panama [103].	Panama	Because of its potential, biofortified rice should be adopted by the agro-industry and other communities.
Study on sensory evaluation of high iron and zinc-rich rice in Cuba [104].	Cuba	Cuba should use biofortified rice since it can help avoid anemia and zinc deficiency.

Table 4.
Past studies on the sensory assessment of biofortified rice within low- and middle-income nations.

Publication	Country	Conclusion
Study on consumer perceptions and impact of negative attributes for folate biofortified rice within China [106].	China	The initial acceptance rate would be cut in half if genetically engineered folate-fortified rice had a negative influence on taste, price, or the environment. Several aspects should be considered when developing biofortified crops.
Study on the potential market for genetically modified rice with health benefits within China [107].	China	There is considerable (segmented) commercial potential for second-generation genetically modified products, especially in the biofortified domain.

Table 5.
Past studies on consumers' acceptance and adoption trends of biofortified rice in low- and middle-income.

about their health advantages are two of the most important variables influencing their acceptability and uptake. According to research, farmers and other stakeholders are prepared to pay a premium for seed production, and after-harvest consumption when they learn about the health benefits of nutrient-rich cultivars (**Table 6**) [112].

To supplement the nutrient-rich varietal adoption, segmented, focused communication methods are required due to the diverse preferences of the respondents being investigated. Because many biofortified varieties have recently progressed from the research and development stage to the dissemination stage, more information on the benefits of biofortified varieties for replacing existing cultivars and bringing dietary changes to consumers should be forthcoming shortly [112].

To secure last-mile distribution, governments, multilateral organizations, farmers, universities, and the commercial sector must form strategic worldwide alliances. Public and private organizations, institutions, and other commercial entities gradually take the lead to assure increased biofortified seed production, enough on-ground delivery, capacity building, and technical assistance to a diverse range of stakeholders, including farmers.

One of the key obstacles to getting biofortified rice varieties broadly adopted and consumed in specific areas is the limitation on the effectiveness of their marketing and geographic spread [113]. There are also further hurdles to marketing nutrient-enriched rice varieties that may limit their widespread acceptance by farmers, other seed value chain actors, and, finally, consumers. Several of them are discussed below.

Publication	Country	Conclusion
Study of consumer's willingness to pay in India in emerging markets for genetically modified foods [108].	India	Most respondents were willing to consume genetically modified foods, and they were willing to pay a considerable premium for golden rice with higher nutritional value.
Study on consumers' willingness to pay for golden rice [109].	Philippines	Golden rice generated through genetic engineering has garnered positive feedback. The marginal impact of positive information versus no information WTP (on willingness to pay) is small for golden rice, whereas negative or two-sided information considerably lowers WTP.
Study on consumers' willingness to pay for genetically modified rice with health benefits within China [110].	China	Nonstudents are less concerned about genetic engineering due to information about folate. Students show a fearful reaction, while in the nonstudent group, contradicting information leads to primacy bias. This demonstrates the need for segmented, targeted biofortification communication techniques.
Study on consumer preferences on folic acid supplementation and folate biofortification within China [111].	China	Positive responses to genetically engineered folate-rich rice support its potential as a supplemental micronutrient intervention.

Table 6.
Past studies on customer willingness to pay for biofortified rice in low- and middle-income nations.

6.1 Challenges in the adoption of nutrient-enriched rice varieties

Most farmers are habituated to growing traditional/existing cultivars due to the assumption of low yields, high input costs, and potential crop loss of biofortified variety. The lack of awareness and empowerment with sufficient information on possible benefits and marketing of nutrient-enriched cultivars to farmers by regional organizations and extension functionaries creates a lengthier transition time for adoption. Most seed business participants, notably the R&D team, make less effort to generate varieties with a solid balance of top desirable features, such as yield, abiotic and biotic tolerance, and nutritional traits. Increased awareness, initiatives, and inclusive, coordinated promotional programs could help to accelerate the growth of nutrient-rich crops. A strengthened focus on R&D should be important for biofortified research. Local organizations struggle to secure enough breeder seeds to produce new varieties due to a lack of government incentives for producers and the inadequate capability of local seed firms. This is due to a lack of resources, capability, and incentives to meet market demand and make R&D investments. Most biofortified rice cultivars, unlike conventional crops, lack differentiating, targeted phenotypic features, such as the desired grain type as well as high yield. As a result, convincing farmers and value chain stakeholders of their greater features over traditional cultivars may be difficult.

Most of the rice growers are smallholders who are extremely price sensitive. Inaccurate pricing information and price changes may discourage farmers from cultivating biofortified cultivars over traditional ones. Nutrient enrichment can sometimes change the color of rice grains or crops. For example, for increased quantities of vitamin A, the ultimate product is orange rather than white rice. Customers may find it difficult to accept and become acclimated to its appearance because of this. Because it can be costly and time-consuming to devise and implement strategies to enhance the shelf life of nutrient-rich rice varieties, the limited shelf life of some biofortified grains may be a barrier to the development of processed products. Processed biofortified rice is being sought after and may fill a niche market. Consumer dynamics will be scaled with various sorts of biofortified rice-based products for consumers.

7. Biofortification in Rice, an impactful strategy for public health

Micronutrients are required for proper growth and development, as well as for optimum health [48, 49]. The primary cause of people's high micronutrient deficits has been attributed to their poor bioavailability after dietary consumption, combined with limited soil micronutrient availability for crop production [114]. Micronutrient malnutrition affects an estimated one-third of the global population due to the dependency on cereal staples for daily nutritional needs along with the limitation to access to diverse nutritional foods and supplements [51]. Global recognition has been acknowledged as an important need for developing a malnutrition mitigation strategy for the SDGs [115]. Previously, numerous strategies were employed to reduce malnutrition, including food fortification, vitamin supplementation, and dietary variety. However, because of high adherence costs and a lack of accessibility and understanding among rural populations, the outcomes were mixed [116]. It has been shown that the biofortification of popular staple crops such as rice is an efficient and relatively low-cost means of alleviating malnutrition. By using this food-based strategy, a targeted population can regulate and avoid micronutrient deficiencies [117–119]. Shortages of iron, zinc, selenium, and iodine create substantial health concerns as well as significant financial losses [120, 121]. Crop production systems should incorporate nutrition-sensitive practices to generate micronutrient-enriched staple foods for the targeted populations [117, 122, 123].

Rice is the most important source of food in terms of energy for more than half of the world's population [124]. It is a significant staple crop in over 40 nations globally, providing at least 20% of daily caloric intake to over 3.5 billion people [1]. However, because milled rice contains fewer nutrients, most marginal groups that rely largely on rice do not have access to a broad mineral supply. Rice biofortification is a long-term and cost-effective solution to the problem of micronutrient deficiency. Rice is a primary food crop for biofortification in many South Asian, Southeast Asian, and African countries [125].

Biofortification has the lowest per capita cost of any intervention, making it particularly accessible and affordable for rural areas [126]. It is critical to breed rice varieties that incorporate beneficial minerals and vitamins to generate a holistically single biofortified rice product. In the fight against hidden hunger, rice biofortification provides a sustainable alternative to chemical food additives, and it should be a top research priority for the most affected countries. Based on the HarvestPlus breeding programs, iron-biofortified rice, for example, is to reach a targeted iron content of roughly 30% over the estimated average requirement of 15 g/g (dry weight) in polished grain [127, 128]. Healthy rice has recently gained popularity and is in high demand in several parts of the world. As a result, to maximize the benefit of establishing nutritional security for public health, we must continue to produce nutritious rice at a rapid rate.

7.1 Policy recommendation

Despite some controversy, such as climate change and the COVID-19 epidemic, the recently concluded United Nations Food Systems Summit resulted in meaningful and revolutionary long-term efforts to achieve zero hunger. These action items were to be used as a measure of achievement to respect, preserve, and fulfill human rights with enough nourishment. Developing resilient food systems from a peace-building perspective can help to promote both long-term food and nutrition security and long-term peace, even if conflict resolution ultimately requires political solutions and societal transformation.

It is important to improve food system resilience to combat the consequences of conflict and environmental concerns while providing food security and nutrition. Moreover, rational decisions are to be made based on a thorough awareness of the situation, with inclusive support and locally driven efforts. Personnel involved in aid, development, and peacekeeping must regularly and methodically assess the current situation globally. Local, national, and international players should all be included in nutritional decision-making. Priority must be given to flexibility, competency, cross-sectoral and long-term planning, and financing. Donors, international entities, nongovernmental organizations, and local seed actors should strive to establish and maintain long-term cross-sectoral linkages. Priorities for funding must be set in a flexible and adaptable manner that considers local perceptions, aspirations, and concerns. Human rights and real community and civil society participation must serve as the foundation of multilateral food governance. The SDGs, the Paris Agreement on Climate Change, and human rights treaties must all be incorporated into food policy activities that prioritize vulnerable people. Governments must seize recent opportunities, such as the United Nations Climate Change Conference (COP 26) and the Tokyo Nutrition for Growth Summit in 2021, to reaffirm the commitment to ending hunger by investing in nutrition and resilience in volatile and conflict-effected environments.

8. Future prospect of biofortified rice

In the current context, biofortification intervention is a promising crop-based strategy for eliminating micronutrient insufficiency. The current biofortification methodology has a considerable research deficit, making general implementation challenging. The mechanisms of nutrient transfer from soil to seed are poorly understood in most food crops, including rice. As a result, a better understanding of the fundamental processes that limit the rate of micronutrient acquisition and translocation in the soil–plant system is required. Before making biofortified crops available to consumers, the safety risks, particularly for genetically modified kinds, must be thoroughly investigated. Another big knowledge gap is in the bioavailability of micronutrients in food grains and the pattern of mineral dispersion in plant systems. It is necessary to study the potential loss of micronutrients during processing as well as the deliberate removal of external tissues. Some of the most recent techniques, such as molecular cytogenetic gene transfer for higher iron and zinc content, uniform mineral distribution in grain to reduce micronutrient loss during postharvest processing, manipulation of phytic acid levels to increase bioavailability, and so on, can play an important role in enriching plant edible parts. We recently discovered that the judicious application of nano-based micronutrient fertilizers may enhance the biofortification process. As a result, it is vital to develop an integrated biofortification approach that can improve human health when eaten through the consumption of micronutrient-fortified food products.

However, there are always questions about the scientific validity of rice biofortification, its potential for adoption by farmers and consumers, its economic sustainability, and production stability before we can utilize it successfully to combat micronutrient deficiencies [129]. Although no significant initiatives to sell nutrient-rich rice have been identified, the purpose of developing biofortified rice is to use it more widely. The discovery of stable transgenic golden rice, a form of rice biofortified with beta-carotene, has resulted in extensive scientific research and development. However, there have been substantial delays in the marketing of golden rice [130]. Rice is the staple food for most of Asia. When considering the commercialization of biofortified rice, it must be kept in mind that the majority of rice is consumed in Asia, and many potential beneficiaries come from developing nations and low-income households. Regulations that prohibit the use of genetically modified rice alongside traditional rice may thus be a practical hurdle for such countries. An interdisciplinary research team comprised of crop science and human nutrition experts must collaborate to generate finished products with desirable nutritional attributes. Biofortified rice will also need to exhibit acceptable sensory and cooking characteristics to gain widespread adoption. Furthermore, it is critical to ensure that the biofortified rice varieties will yield at the required level and will be resistant to biotic and abiotic problems. The biofortification program for rice is being effectively implemented in several nations because of enhanced marketing, agricultural policy, nutrition education, and public awareness campaigns. As a result, additional deliberate efforts toward the development of biofortified crops along with suitable agronomic management practices must be adopted in the future to mitigate micronutrient deficiency in humans and provide food and nutritional security.

9. Summary

Malnutrition has a global impact on human learning ability, immune system function, and physical and mental development. Hidden hunger, often known as micronutrient deficiency, is a major global concern. The nonavailability of minerals and vitamins is expected to grow more in the future, and biofortification is on the path to the establishment as a feasible treatment. For greater human health, the interplay of iron, zinc, and vitamin must be synergistic and increase mineral bioavailability. This intrinsic "synergistic impact" stimulates plant breeders to combine these nutrients in the future to generate improved biofortified rice, which may be considered an advancement over other traditional approaches. Rice is being biofortified with additional vitamins and minerals to address hidden hunger. Biofortification of rice with folic acid (or folate), thiamin, riboflavin, niacin, pantothenic acid, pyridoxine, biotin, vitamin B12, ascorbic acid, vitamin D, and vitamin E is ongoing [131]. Rice biofortification should be a major focus of research and development efforts in affected countries. Researchers of biofortified rice, policymakers, stakeholders, and philanthropists should focus on policies that directly benefit rice consumers in affected countries, such as the public-private partnership model in agri-biotech research, "freedom to operate" biofortified rice varieties developed by private companies, area-specific production, better storage facilities, international rice distribution policies, and raising awareness. Furthermore, the COVID-19 pandemic, a current global health emergency, as well as several illnesses caused by micronutrient deficiency, have drawn attention to the utility of biofortified crops as a viable and cost-effective method of providing important micronutrients to billions of people worldwide. These biofortification strategies will assist those who are vulnerable in becoming more resilient to future shocks to food and income systems caused by unfavorable causes such as prospective pandemics and natural disasters. Governments should therefore encourage the widespread and augmented adoption of biofortified staple crops, particularly rice, by providing financial incentives. There has been great progress in this field, and with more planned studies and robust laws, rice biofortification may see considerable success in the coming years. As a result, biofortified rice has significant potential for addressing the issue of micronutrient insufficiency, with excellent prospects for its adoption and influence in assuring the nutritional security of the world's population by reaching the unreached.

Acknowledgements

The authors acknowledge the efforts of Mr. Sarvesh Shukla (Agricultural Officer, IRRI-SARC) and Mr. Rabindra Moharana (Research Technician IRRI-SARC) in assisting during the preparation of the manuscript.

Author details

Kuntal Das[1*], Priyabrata Roy[2] and Raj Kumar Singh Tiwari[1]

1 BTC College of Agriculture and Research Station, Indira Gandhi Krishi Vishwavidyalaya, Bilaspur, Chhattisgarh, India

2 Department of Molecular Biology and Biotechnology, University of Kalyani, Kalyani, West Bengal, India

*Address all correspondence to: kdas_mail@yahoo.com

References

[1] FAO. The Future of Food and Agriculture: Trends and Challenges. Rome: Food and Agriculture Organization of the United Nations; 2013

[2] Arouna A, Fatognon IA, Saito K, Futakuchi K. Moving toward rice self-sufficiency in sub-Saharan Africa by 2030: Lessons learned from 10 years of the Coalition for African Rice Development. World Development Perspectives. 2021;**21**:100-291

[3] Sautter C, Poletti S, Zhang P, Gruissem W. Biofortification of essential nutritional compounds and trace elements in rice and cassava. Proceedings of the Nutrition Society. 2006;**65**(2):153-159

[4] Han X, Ding S, Lu J, Li Y. Global, regional, and national burdens of common micronutrient deficiencies from 1990 To 2019: A secondary trend analysis based on the global burden of disease 2019 study. EClinical Medicine. 2022;**44**:101-299

[5] Caballero B. Global patterns of child health: The role of nutrition. Annals of Nutrition and Metabolism. 2002;**46**(Suppl. 1):3-7

[6] Ruel-Bergeron JC, Stevens GA, Sugimoto JD, Roos FF, Ezzati M, Black RE, et al. Global update and trends of hidden hunger, 1995-2011: The hidden hunger index. PLoS One. 2015;**10**(12):e0143497

[7] Bouis HE, Welch RM. Biofortification-a sustainable agricultural strategy for reducing micronutrient malnutrition in the global south. Crop Science. 2010;**50**:S-20

[8] Saltzman A, Birol E, Bouis HE, Boy E, De Moura FF, Islam Y. Pfeiffer WH. Biofortification: Progress toward a more nourishing future. Global Food Security. 2013;**2**(1):9-17.

[9] Saltzman A, Birol E, Bouis HE. Biofortification: Progress toward a more nourishing future. Global Food Security. 2013;**2**:9-17

[10] Datta S, Bouis HE. Application of biotechnology to improving the nutritional quality of rice. Food and Nutrition Bulletin. 2000;**21**(4):451-456

[11] WHO. The State of Food Security and Nutrition in the World 2021: Transforming Food Systems for Food Security, Improved Nutrition and Affordable Healthy Diets for all. Food & Agriculture Org; 2021

[12] Lowe NM. The global challenge of hidden hunger: Perspectives from the field. Proceedings of the Nutrition Society. 2021;**80**(3):283-289

[13] Saltzman A, Birol E, Wiesman D, Prasai N, Yohannes Y, Menon P, et al. 2014 Global Hunger Index: The Challenge of Hidden Hunger. International Food Policy Research Institute. Bonn, Washington, D.C., Dublin. 2014

[14] Micha R, Mannar V, Afshin A, Allemandi L, Baker P, Battersby J, et al. In: Behrman N, editor. Global Nutrition Report: Action on Equity to End Malnutrition. Bristol, UK: Development Initiatives; 2020

[15] Popkin BM, Corvalan C, Grummer-Strawn LM. Dynamics of the double burden of malnutrition and the changing nutrition reality. The Lancet. 2020;**395**(10217):65-74

[16] Moniz CS, Carvalho R, Prazeres S, Limbert E, Mendes I, César R. Efficacy of

a salt iodization program on iodine status and intakes in school children of São Miguel Island, Azores. Portugal. European Thyroid Journal. 2021;**10**(2):109-113

[17] FAO, IFAD, UNICEF, WFP, WHO. The State of Food Security and Nutrition in the World 2021. Transforming Food Systems for Food Security, Improved Nutrition and Affordable Healthy Diets for all. Rome: FAO; 2021

[18] Weisstaub G, Araya M, Hill A, Uauy R. Childhood malnutrition: Prevention and control at the national level. In: Nutrition in Pediatrics. 4th ed. Hamilton, Canada: BC Decker; 2003

[19] Black RE. Global distribution and disease burden related to micronutrient deficiencies. In: International Nutrition: Achieving Millennium Goals and beyond. Vol. 78. Basel: Karger Publishers; 2014. pp. 21-28

[20] Allen LH. Iron supplements: Scientific issues concerning efficacy and implications for research and programs. The Journal of Nutrition. 2002;**132**(4):813S-819S

[21] WHO. Global Nutrition Targets 2025: Stunting Policy Brief. World Health Organization; 2014

[22] Hoddinott J, Alderman H, Behrman JR, Haddad L, Horton S. The economic rationale for investing in stunting reduction. Maternal & Child Nutrition. 2013;**9**:69-82

[23] Biesalski HK. Strategies to combat hidden hunger. In Hidden hunger. Heidelberg: Berlin, Heidelberg; 2013. pp. 207-245

[24] Diamond J. Evolution, consequences and future of plant and animal domestication. Nature. 2002;**418**:700-707

[25] Doebley JF, Gaut BS, Smith BD. The molecular genetics of crop domestication. Cell. 2006;**127**(7):1309-1321

[26] Larson G, Fuller DQ. The evolution of animal domestication. Annual Revolution of Ecology, Evolution and Systematics. 2014;**66**:115-136

[27] Fuller DQ. Pathways to Asian civilizations: Tracing the origins and spread of rice and rice cultures. Rice. 2011;**4**:78-92

[28] Sweeny M, McCouch S. The complex history of the domestication of rice. Annals of Botany. 2007;**100**:951-957

[29] Bellon MR, Dulloo E, Sardos J, Thormann I, Burdon JJ. In situ conservation-harnessing natural and human derived evolutionary forces to ensure future crop adaptation. Evolutionary Applications. 2017;**10**(10):965-977

[30] Deb D. Folk rice varieties, traditional knowledge and nutritional security in South Asia. In: Poyyamoli G, editor. Agroecology, Ecosystems, and Sustainability in the Tropics. New Delhi: Studera Press; 2017. pp. 117-134

[31] Debal D. Food sovereignty: Opposing the enclosure of land, seeds and knowledge commons. In: Mentschel S, editor. Can Hunger be Defeated? Yoda Press. New Delhi; 2019. pp. 1-48

[32] Sen Gupta S, Baksi A, Roy P, Deb D, Pradeep T. Unusual accumulation of silver in the aleurone layer of an Indian rice (*Oryza sativa*) landrace and sustainable extraction of the metal. ACS Sustainable Chemistry & Engineering. 2017;**5**(9):8310-8315

[33] Sulochana S, Meyyappan RM, Singaravadivel K. Phytochemical screening and GC-MS analysis of Garudan samba traditional rice variety. International Journal of Agriculture and Environmental Research. 2016;**2**(4):44-47

[34] Rahman S, Sharma MP, Sahai S. Nutritional and medicinal values of indigenous rice varieties. Indian Journal of Traditional Knowledge. 2006;**5**(4):454-458

[35] Gul K, Yousuf B, Singh AK, Singh P, Wani AA. Rice bran: Nutritional values and its emerging potential for development of functional food-A review. Bioactive Carbohydrates and Dietary Fibre. 2015;**6**(1):24-30

[36] Ashraf AM, Lokanadan S. Effect of seedling age on productivity and profitability in traditional rice landraces. ORYZA-An International Journal of Rice. 2022;**59**(1):113-125

[37] Deb D, Sengupta S, Pradeep T. A profile of heavy metals in rice (Oryza sativa ssp. indica) landraces. Current Science., 2015;**109**(3):407-409

[38] Ranilla LG, Kwon YI, Apostolidis E, Shetty K. Phenolic compounds, antioxidant activity and in vitro inhibitory potential against key enzymes relevant for hyperglycemia and hypertension of commonly used medicinal plants, herbs and spices in Latin America. Bioresource Technology. 2010;**101**(12):4676-4689

[39] Deepa G, Singh V, Naidu KA. Nutrient composition and physicochemical properties of Indian medicinal rice–Njavara. Food Chemistry. 2008;**106**(1):165-171

[40] Roy P. Importance of traditional rice landraces as nutraceutical foods. In: Sinha A et al., editors. Folk Rice Diversity of Eastern India: Hope for the Future Food Security. New Delhi: Innovative Publication; 2019. pp. 123-136

[41] Joseph J, Francies RM, Zachariah G, AV SK. Characterisation of navara (*Oryza sativa* L.) a traditional medicinal rice of Kerala for qualitative traits. Indian. Journal of Agricultural Research. 2007;**41**(4):267-271

[42] Srinivasa D, Raman A, Meena P, Chitale G, Marwahat A, Jainani KJ. Glycaemic index (GI) of an Indian branded thermally treated basmati rice variety: A multi centric study. The Journal of the Association of Physicians of India. 2013;**61**(10):716-720

[43] Umadevi M, Pushpa R, Sampathkumar KP, Bhowmik D. Rice-traditional medicinal plant in India. Journal of Pharmacognosy and Phytochemistry. 2012;**1**(1):6-12

[44] Champagne ET, Wood DF, Juliano BO, Bechtel DB. The rice grain and its gross composition. In: Champagne ET, editor. Rice Chemistry and Technology. Chapter 4. Minneapolis, MN: American Association of Cereal Chemists Press; 2004. pp. 93-96

[45] Dexter PB. Rice Fortification for Developing Countries. Washington, DC, USA: OMNI/USAID; 1998

[46] Luh BS. Rice-I: Production. 2nd ed. New York, NY, USA: Van Nostrand Reinhold; 1991

[47] Masuda H, Usuda K, Kobayashi T, Ishimaru Y, Kakei Y, Takahashi M, et al. Overexpression of the barley nicotianamine synthase gene HvNAS1 increases iron and zinc concentrations in rice grains. Rice. 2009;**2**:155-166

[48] Maret W. Zinc in cellular regulation: The nature and significance of "zinc signals". International Journal of Molecular Sciences. 2017;**18**:2285

[49] Palanog AD, Calayugan MIC, Descalsota-Empleo GI. Zinc and iron nutrition status in the Philippines

population and local soils. Frontiers in Nutrition. 2019;**6**:81

[50] Caulfield LE, Richard SA, Rivera JA. Stunting, wasting, and micronutrient deficiency disorders. In: Jamison DT, Breman JG, Measham AR, et al., editors. Disease Control Priorities in Developing Countries. 2nd ed. Washington, DC: The International Bank for Reconstruction and Development/The World Bank; 2006

[51] Ritchie H, Reay D, Higgins P. Quantifying, projecting, and addressing India's hidden hunger. Frontier in Sustainability Food System. 2018;**2**:11

[52] Khush GS, Lee S, Cho JI, Jeon JS. Biofortification of crops for reducing malnutrition. Plant Biotechnol Rep. 2012;**6**:195-202

[53] Bouis HE. Enrichment of food staples through plant breeding: A new strategy for fighting micronutrient malnutrition. Nutrition. 2000;**16**:701-704

[54] Hirschi KD. Nutrient biofortification of food crops. Annual Review of Nutrition. 2009;**29**:401-421

[55] Zhu C, Naqvi S, Gomez-Galera S, Pelacho AM, Capell T, Christou P. Transgenic strategies for the nutritional enhancement of plants. Trends in Plant Science. 2007;**12**:548-555

[56] Beyer P, Al-Babili S, Ye X, Lucca P, Schaub P, Welsch R. Golden rice: Introducing the β-carotene biosynthesis pathway into rice endosperm by genetic engineering to defeat vitamin A deficiency. The Journal of Nutrition. 2002;**132**(3):506S-510S

[57] Datta K, Baisakh N, Oliva N, Torrizo L, Abrigo E, Tan J. Bioengineered 'golden' Indica rice cultivars with beta-carotene metabolism in the endosperm with hygromycin and mannose selection systems. Plant Biotechnology Journal, 2003;1:81-90

[58] Paine JA, Shipton CA, Chaggar S, Howells RM, Kennedy MJ, Vernon G. Improving the nutritional value of golden rice through increased pro-vitamin a content. Nature Biotechnology. 2005;**23**:482-487

[59] Ye X, Al-Babili S, Kloti A, Zhang J, Lucca P, Beyer P. Engineering the provitamin a (β-carotene) biosynthetic pathway into (carotenoids-free) rice endosperm. Science. 2000;**287**:303-305

[60] Blancquaert D, Van Daele J, Strobbe S, Kiekens F, Storozhenko S, de Steur H. Improving folate (vitamin B9) stability in biofortified rice through metabolic engineering. Nature Biotechnology. 2015;**33**:1076-1078

[61] Storozhenko S, De Brouwer V, Volckaert M, Navarrete O, Blancquaert D, Zhang GF. Folate fortification of rice by metabolic engineering. Nature Biotechnology. 2007;**25**(11):1277-1279

[62] Lee S, Kim YS, Jeon US, Kim YK, Schjoerring JK, An G. Activation of rice nicotinamine synthase 2 (OsNAS2) enhances iron availability for biofortification. Molecular Cell. 2012;**33**:269-275

[63] Lee TTT, Wang MMC, Hou RCW, Chen LJ, Su RC, Wang CS. Enhanced methionine and cysteine levels in transgenic rice seeds by the accumulation of sesame 2S albumin. Bioscience, Biotechnology, and Biochemistry. 2003;**67**:1699-1705

[64] Lucca P, Hurrell R, Potrykus I. Fighting iron deficiency anemia with iron-rich rice. Journal of the American College of Nutrition. 2002;**21**:184-190

[65] Masuda H, Ishimaru Y, Aung MS, Kobayashi T, Kakei Y, Takahashi M. Iron biofortification in rice by the introduction of multiple genes involved in iron nutrition. Scientific Reports. 2012;**2**:534

[66] Masuda H, Kobayashi T, Ishimaru Y, Takahashi M, Aung MS, Nakanishi H. Iron-biofortification in rice by the introduction of three barley genes participated in mugineic acid biosynthesis with soybean ferritin gene. Front. Plant Science. 2013;**4**:132

[67] Takahashi M, Nakanishi H, Kawasaki S. Enhanced tolerance of rice to low iron availability in alkaline soils using barley nicotianamine aminotransferase genes. Nature Biotechnology. 2001;**19**:466-469

[68] Trijatmiko K, Duenas C, Tsakirpaloglou N, Torrizo L, Arines FM, Adeva C. Biofortified indica rice attains iron and zinc nutrition dietary targets in the field. Scientific Reports. 2016;**6**:197-192

[69] Vasconcelos M, Datta K, Oliva N, Khalekuzzaman M, Torrizo L, Krishnan S. Enhanced iron and zinc accumulation in transgenic rice with the ferritin gene. Plant Science. 2003;**164**:371-378

[70] Wirth J, Poletti S, Aeschlimann B, Yakandawala N, Drosse B, Osorio S. Rice endosperm iron biofortification by targeted and synergistic action of nicotianamine synthase and ferritin. Plant Biotechnology Journal. 2009;**7**:631-644

[71] Hurrell R, Egli I. Iron bioavailability and dietary reference values. The American Journal of Clinical Nutrition. 2010;**91**:1461-1467

[72] Lee S, An G. Over-expression of OsIRT1 leads to increased iron and zinc accumulations in rice. Plant, Cell & Environment. 2009;**32**:408-416

[73] Masuda H, Suzuki M, Morikawa KC, Kobayashi T, Nakanishi H, Takahashi M. Increase in iron and zinc concentrations in rice grains via the introduction of barley genes involved in phytosiderophore synthesis. Rice. 2008;**1**:100-108

[74] Katsube T, Kurisaka N, Ogawa M, Maruyama N, Ohtsuka R, Utsumi S. Accumulation of soybean glycinin and its assembly with the glutelins in rice. Plant Physiology. 1999;**120**:1063-1073

[75] Lee SI, Kim HU, Lee YH, Suh SC, Lim YP, Lee HY. Constitutive and seed-specific expression of a maize lysine-feedback-insensitive dihydrodipicolinate synthase gene leads to increased free lysine levels in rice seeds. Molecular Breeding. 2001;**8**:75-84

[76] Wakasa K, Hasegawa H, Nemoto H, Matsuda F, Miyazawa H, Tozawa Y. High-level tryptophan accumulation in seeds of transgenic rice and its limited effects on agronomic traits and seed metabolite profile. Journal of Experimental Botany. 2006;**57**:3069-3078

[77] Yang QQ, Zhang CQ, Chan ML, Zhao DS, Chen JZ, Wang Q. Biofortification of rice with the essential amino acid lysine: Molecular characterization, nutritional evaluation, and field performance. Journal of Experimental Botany. 2016;**67**(14):4285-4296

[78] Zhou Y, Cai H, Xiao J, Li X, Zhang Q, Lian X. Over-expression of aspartate aminotransferase genes in rice resulted in altered nitrogen metabolism and increased amino acid content in seeds. Theoretical and Applied Genetics. 2009;**118**:1381-1390

[79] Anai T, Koga M, Tanaka H, Kinoshita T, Rahman SM, Takagi Y. Improvement of rice (*Oryza sativa* L.)

seed oil quality through introduction of a soybean microsomal omega-3 fatty acid desaturase gene. Plant Cell Reports. 2003;**21**(10):988-992

[80] Ogo Y, Ozawa K, Ishimaru T, Murayama T, Takaiwa F. Transgenic rice seed synthesizing diverse flavonoids at high levels: A new platform for flavonoid production with associated health benefits. Plant Biotechnology Journal. 2013;**11**:734-746

[81] Shin YM, Park HJ, Yim SD, Baek NI, Lee CH, An G. Transgenic rice lines expressing maize C1 and R-S regulatory genes produce various flavonoids in the endosperm. Plant Biotechnology Journal. 2006;**4**:303-315

[82] Liu Q, Wang Z, Chen X, Cai X, Tang S, Yu H. Stable inheritance of the antisense waxy gene in transgenic rice with reduced amylose level and improved quality. Transgenic Research. 2003;**12**(1):71-82

[83] Itoh K, Ozaki H, Okada K, Hori H, Takeda Y, Mitsui T. Introduction of wx transgene into rice wx mutants leads to both high- and low-amylose rice. Plant & Cell Physiology. 2003;**44**(5):473-480

[84] Wei C, Zhang J, Chen Y, Zhou W, Xu B, Wang Y. Physicochemical properties and development of wheat large and small starch granules during endosperm development. Acta Physiologiae Plantarum. 2010;**32**:905-916

[85] Nandi S, Suzuki YA, Huang J, Yalda D, Pham P, Wu L. Expression of human lactoferrin in transgenic rice grains for the application in infant formula. Plant Science. 2002;**163**:713-722

[86] Fang Y, Wang L, Xin Z, Zhao L, An X, Hu Q. Effect of foliar application of zinc, selenium, and iron fertilizers on nutrients concentration and yield of rice grain in China. Journal of Agricultural and Food Chemistry. 2008;**6**(56):2079-2084

[87] He W, Shohag MJ, Wei Y, Feng Y, Yang X. Iron concentration, bioavailability, and nutritional quality of polished rice affected by different forms of foliar iron fertilizer. Food Chemistry. 2013;**141**(4):4122-4126

[88] Wei Y, Shohag MJ, Yang X. Biofortification and bioavailability of rice grain zinc as affected by different forms of foliar zinc fertilization. PLoS One. 2012;**7**(9):e45428

[89] Yuan L, Wu L, Yang C, Quin LV. Effects of iron and zinc foliar applications on rice plants and their grain accumulation and grain nutritional quality. Journal of the Science of Food and Agriculture. 2013;**93**(2):254-261

[90] Boonchuay P, Cakmak I, Rerkasem B, Prom-U-Thai C. Effect of different foliar zinc application at different growth stages on seed zinc concentration and its impact on seedling vigor in rice. Soil Science & Plant Nutrition. 2013;**59**(2):180-188

[91] Guo JX, Feng XM, Hu XY, Tian GL. Effects of soil zinc availability, nitrogen fertilizer rate and zinc fertilizer application method on zinc biofortification of rice. The Journal of Agricultural Science. 2016;**154**(4):584-597

[92] Mabesa RL, Impa SM, Grewal D, Beebout SEJ. Contrasting grain-Zn response of biofortification rice (Oryza sativa L.) breeding lines to foliar Zn application. Field Crops Research. 2013;**149**:223-233

[93] Ram H, Rashid A, Zhang W, Duarte AP, Phattarakul N, Simunji S. Biofortification of wheat, rice and common bean by applying foliar zinc fertilizer along with pesticides in seven countries. Plant and Soil. 2016;**1**(403):389-401

[94] Shivay YS, Kumar D, Prasad R, Ahlawat IPS. Relative yield and zinc uptake by rice from zinc sulphate and zinc oxide coatings onto urea. Nutrition Cycling Agroecosystem. 2008;**80**(2):181-188

[95] Giacosa A, Faliva MA, Perna S, Minoia C, Ronchi A, Rondanelli M. Selenium fortification of an Italian rice cultivar via foliar fertilization with sodium selenate and its effects on human serum selenium levels and on erythrocyte glutathione peroxidase activity. Nutrients. 2014;**6**(3):1251-1261

[96] Liu K, Gu Z. Selenium accumulation in different brown rice cultivars and its distribution in fractions. Journal of Agricultural and Food Chemistry. 2009;**57**(2):695-700

[97] Premarathna L, McLaughlin MJ, Kirby JK, Hettiarachchi GM, Stacey S, Chittleborough DJ. Selenate-enriched urea granules are a highly effective fertilizer for selenium biofortification of paddy rice grain. Journal of Agricultural and Food Chemistry. 2012;**60**(23):6037-6044

[98] Xu J, Hu Q. Effect of foliar application of selenium on the antioxidant activity of aqueous and ethanolic extracts of selenium-enriched rice. Journal of Agricultural and Food Chemistry. 2004;**52**(6):1759-1763

[99] Ekin B, Jen F, Destan A. Biofortification: The evidence. Harvest Plus Newsletter. Washington, DC: International Food Policy Research Institute (IFPRI); 2021. Available from: https://www.harvestplus.org/wpcontent/uploads/2021/12/Biofortification_The-Evidence.pdf

[100] Peters DH, Tran NT, Adam T. Implementation Research in Health: A Practical Guide. Geneva, Switzerland: World Health Organization; 2013

[101] De Bree A. Acceptability of Zinc Fortified Rice by Women in Rural Chuzhou District, China. Wageningen, the Netherlands: Wageningen University; 2009

[102] Montecinos KL, Godoy JA, Centeno PM. Evaluación sensorial de arroz (Oryza sativa) variedad azucena en la región autónoma del Atlántico Norte en Nicaragua. Perspect en Nutr Humana. 2011;**13**:135-146

[103] Vergara O, Buitrago IC, De Caballero EV. Evaluación sensorial de arroz biofortificade, variedad IDIAP Santa Cruz 11, en granjas autosostenibles del patronato de Nutrición en la provincia de Coclé, Panama. Perspect en Nutr. Humana. 2011;**13**:147-160

[104] Padrón V, Crestelo E, Caraballo R. Preferencia y aceptabilidad de la variedad de arroz IACuba 30 con alto contenido de hierro y zinc por mujeres gestantes en Cuba—ProQuest. Perspective in Nutritional Humana. 2011;**13**:123-134

[105] Birol E, Meenakshi JV, Oparinde A. Developing country consumers' acceptance of biofortified foods: A synthesis. Food Security. 2015;**7**:555-568

[106] De Steur H, Blancquaert D, Gellynck X. How negative product attributes alter consumer perceptions of folate biofortified rice in a high risk region of China. International Journal of Biotechnology. 2013;**12**:269-287

[107] De Steur HD, Liqun G, Van Der Straeten D. The potential market for GM rice with health benefits in a Chinese high-risk region. Journal of Food Products Marketing. 2015;**21**:231-243

[108] Deodhar SY, Chern WS. Emerging markets for GM foods: a study of consumer's willingness to pay in India emerging markets for GM foods:

an Indian perspective on consumer understanding and willingness to pay. In: Paper presented at: American Agricultural Economics Association Annual Meeting. Orlando; 2008

[109] Depositario DPT, Nayga RM, Wu X Jr. Effects of information on consumers' willingness to pay for golden rice. Asian. The Econometrics Journal. 2009;**23**:457-476

[110] De Steur HD, Buysse J, Feng S. Role of information on consumers' willingness-to-pay for genetically-modified rice with health benefits: An application to China. Asian. The Econometrics Journal. 2013;**27**:391-408

[111] De Steur H, Feng S, Xiaoping S. Consumer preferences for micronutrient strategies in China. A comparison between folic acid supplementation and folate biofortification. Public Health Nutrition. 2014;**17**:1410-1420

[112] Talsma EF, Melse-Boonstra A, Brouwer ID. Acceptance and adoption of biofortified crops in low- and middle-income countries: A systematic review. Nutrition Reviews. 2017;**75**(10):798-829

[113] Gilligan DO, Kumar N, McNiven S. IFPRI Discussion Paper 01353: Bargaining Power and Biofortification: The Role of Gender in Adoption of Orange Sweet Potato in Uganda. Washington, DC: International Food Policy and Research Institute (IFPRI); 2014

[114] Welch RM, Graham RD, Cakmak I. Linking agricultural production practices to improving human nutrition and health. In: Expert Paper Written for ICN2 Second International Conference on Nutrition Preparatory Technical Meeting. Rome, Italy; 2013. pp. 13-15

[115] Hanieh S, High H, Boulton J. Nutrition justice: Uncovering invisible pathways to malnutrition. Frontiers in Endocrinology. 2020;**11**:150

[116] Bouis HE. An overview of the landscape and approach for biofortifcation in Africa. African Journal of Food Agriculture Nutrition and Development. 2017;**17**(2):11848-11864

[117] Bouis HE, Saltzman A. Improving nutrition through biofortification: a review of evidence from HarvestPlus through 2016. Global Food Security. 2003;**12**:49-58

[118] Szymlek-Gay EA, Ferguson EL, Heath AL, Gray AR, Gibson RS. Food-based strategies improve iron status in toddlers: A randomized controlled trial. The American Journal of Clinical Nutrition. 2009;**90**:1541-1551

[119] Torheim LE, Ferguson EL, Penrose K, Arimond M. Women in resource-poor settings are at risk of inadequate intakes of multiple micronutrients. The Journal of Nutrition. 2010;**140**:2051-2058

[120] Bailey RL, West KP Jr, Black RE. The epidemiology of global micronutrient deficiencies. Annals of Nutrition & Metabolism. 2015;**66**(Suppl. 2):22-33

[121] Harding KL, Aguayo VM, Webb P. Hidden hunger in South Asia: A review of recent trends and persistent challenges. Public Health Nutrition. 2018;**21**:785-795

[122] Cakmak I, Kutman UB. Agronomic biofortification of cereals with zinc: A review. European Journal of Soil Science. 2018;**69**:172-180

[123] Jha AB, Warkentin TD. Biofortification of pulse crops: Status and future perspectives. Plants. 2020;**9**:73

[124] Gross BL, Zhao Z. Archaeological and genetic insights into the origins

of domesticated rice. Proceedings of the National Academy of Sciences. 2014;**111**(17):61-90

[125] Siwela M, Pillay K, Govender L, Lottering S. Biofortifed crops for combating hidden hunger in South Africa: Availability, acceptability, micronutrient retention and bioavailability. Food. 2020;**9**(6):815

[126] Ma G, Jin Y, Li Y, Zhai F, Kok FJ, Jacobsen E, et al. Iron and zinc defciencies in China: What is a feasible and cost-effective strategy? Public Health Nutrition. 2008;**11**:632-638

[127] Oliva N, Chadha-Mohanty P, Poletti S, Abrigo E, Atienza G, Torrizo L. Large-scale production and evaluation of marker-free indica rice IR64 expressing phytoferritin genes. Molecular Breeding. 2014;**33**(1):23-37

[128] Vasconcelos MW, Gruissem W. Iron BNK. Biofortification in the 21st century: Setting realistic targets, overcoming obstacles, and new strategies for healthy nutrition. Current Opinion in Biotechnology. 2017;**44**(1):8-15

[129] Nestel P, Bouis HE, Meenakshi JV, Pfeiffer W. Biofortification of staple food crops. The Journal of Nutrition. 2006;**136**(4):1064-1067

[130] Potrykus I. From the concept of totipotency to biofortified cereals. Annual Review of Plant Biology. 2015;**32**:1-22

[131] Ghosh S, Datta K, Datta SK. Rice vitamins. In: Bao J, editor. Rice Chemistry and Technology. 1st ed. Amsterdam, The Netherlands: Elsevier Inc.; 2019. pp. 195-220